Ear Acupuncture

The complete text
by the Nanking army
ear acupuncture
team

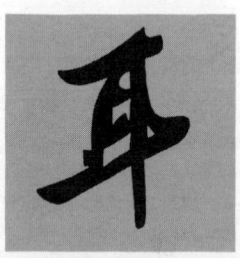

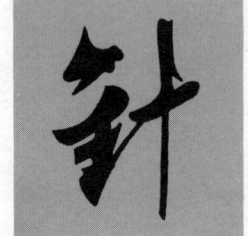

Ear
Acupuncture

Translated by
Helena L. Huang, Ph.D.

With an Introduction and an Afterword by
Dr. Frank Warren

Rodale Press, Inc. Book Division
Emmaus, Pennsylvania 18049

Traditional Chinese medicine is a great treasure house which ought to be explored and further enriched.

Mao Tse-tung

In medical and health work priority must be given to the countryside.

Mao Tse-tung

Translation of the Chinese text *Erh chen* compiled by an ear acupuncture team of the Nanking army and published in December 1972 by the People Publishing House, Shanghai, China.

Printed in the United States of America on recycled paper

Book design by Repro-Art Service

First Printing — March 1974
Second Printing — October 1975
B-659

International Standard Book Number 0-87857-078-0

Library of Congress Card Number 73-21131

Library of Congress Cataloging in Publication Data

Translation of Erh chen.
1. Acupuncture. [DNLM: 1. Acupuncture.
2. Ear. WB369 N182e 1974]
RM184.E7413   615'.892   73-21131
ISBN 0-87857-078-0

iv

Table of Contents

Introduction

With the recent upsurge of interest and research in general acupuncture in the United States (although it has been widely known throughout Europe and the Eastern worlds), it was inevitable that the forum of attention should turn to ear acupuncture.

What is ear acupuncture? How did it evolve? What is its relationship to the total field? These questions are amply answered in the following volume. Some reserve of course is necessary so that our perspectives may not be overwhelmed by the enthusiasm of the writers, nor undermined by its obvious propaganda for the political system of Chairman Mao.

The external ear is a curious organ, considered by some to be nothing more than a vestigial replica of the pinna in animals, where it served a much more functional purpose.

In some civilizations the human external ear was considered an organ of punishment, a tribute to its rich nerve supply. More recently, as in the notorious Getty case, we have seen it become an intrument of ransom, in a revival of the "banditti" days.

By many workers in the field, ear acupuncture is considered the ultimate in treatment modalities. It was presumed that one would first learn the acupuncture of the body points and then go on to its more esoteric derivative, auriculo (ear) therapy. Lately, it has become obvious to investigators that the ear points can act not only as an extremely powerful augmentation of the body points, but also on their own. In fact, a separation of these two techniques would be akin to the concept which existed for many years in popular medicine concerning the "psycho" and the "soma". It was customary 50 years ago to separate diseases of the mind and of the body. However, today we know there are a great many afflictions which are considered psychosomatic and recognize that factors of mind and body contribute equally to their existence. The same thing applies with ear and body acupuncture as far as treatment is concerned. Both ear and body points should be used concomitantly or individually, as the conditions dictate, not as parts of a separate mechanism, but as interrelated modalities. I am quite sure not every one will agree with this viewpoint, especially purists. However this is what has worked for me and many associates here in clinical practice in the United States.

Juding by the effects of its penetration, it seems fairly apparent that the skin is not the simple histologically-layered, inactive bag depicted in most medical texts. As a result of early impressions, a majority of students carry away with them an erroneous idea of the skin. This is due for a change, thanks to the new Oriental and European thinking. They believe, if one is to understand modern acupuncture, that our conception of the physiology and anatomy of the skin must be radicalized to account for heretofore poorly described phenomena such as microcurrents, changing areas of diminished resistance, shifting areas of increased potential, magnetic layer attraction, and other electrophysiological facts or artifacts which can be demonstrated in the living skin.

The histologists describe seven layers of cells in the epidermis, the dermis, and various layers of subcutaneous fat and connective tissue. Physiologists discuss some important functions in terms of thermal regulation and excretion, but little or no mention is made of the bio-electromagnetic fields within the skin, constantly in play, constantly undergoing ionic atmospheric bombardment. In fact, it is not inconceivable that this ionic bombardment (e.g. in a heavily ionized room) may be partly responsible for the first gasp of life, since it can be postulated to be caused by external as well as biochemical stimulation. This could be conceptualized into an ionic-humoral-chemical cause for the infant's first breath. In any case, the human skin, developing as it does from the ectodermal layer, can be demonstrated to be more than just a baggy envelope, holding together the contents of the body. In fact, in some investigator's opinions, it is probably as important an organ as any of the internal viscera.

In the ear, the skin varies from being stretched to a minimum thickness over cartilage, to a maximum where it has many layers and is relatively insensitive (in lobule). This fact is definitely of paramount interest in judging the effects of auricular stimulation; just as the ear is one of the most important areas for studying some of the variations of the skin. And ear acupuncture then becomes the widely varied yet phenomenally accurate subspecialty we know it to be.

It is difficult to accept the idea that there are approximately 200 points in the ear, each one relatively small, yet each capable of producing a response to stimulation. (The average practitioner, hard-pressed to accommodate for acupuncture to begin with, finds himself in even deeper intellectual waters when confronted with this idea.)

Nevertheless, there are physiologic and therapeutic phenomena in this startling category that he has already accepted, unbeknownst to him. If he is a student of medical history, he must surely be aware of the fact that the empiric tradition of cauterization of the external ear for the treatment of sciatic neuralgia was prevalent in the Mediterranean Basin, practiced mostly by Egyptians; in the East by Persians; in Africa, and in later years by Greek, French, and Italians. Medieval and Renaissance artists have attempted to depict this technique, indicating a point on the anthelix which is replicated later in modern books. So that apparently the ear points, as well as the body points, have survived in antiquity.

If we consider ourselves descendants of Hippocratic medicine, then we must certainly know that the great master also prescribed a treatment of the painful condition we today call sciatica. His recommendation, similarly, was cauterization of the ear, although the area prescribed was not the one used by most ear accupuncture enthusiasts of our times. Nevertheless, the ideology is identical.

In the Summation chapter, you will read more of the embryology of the ear and why one finds this close relationship between the points of ear stimulation and the body responses. Although the two are ostensibly distant and unconnected by the known neurologic foundation we learned in our professional schools, the results are indisputable. There must therefore be some connection of which we know little, but which will be discovered in years to come.

Suffice it to say that for the now, the embryology supplies the missing link which enables us to bridge the gap between what we see and what we know as it concerns ear acupuncture. The French clinician, Paul Nogier, has been an assiduous worker in this field for the past twenty years. Today, at an age when most physicians would be retiring, he is still extremely active in his clinic as well as in his school, benevolently directing dozens of students who flock to his study in Lyon from all parts of Europe and the Americas. Between the French school of Auriculo-Therapy and the Chinese schools of ear acupuncture, a great deal more will be learned in future years about the treatment of the human body with needles.

Frank Z. Warren, M.D.

New York, N.Y.   Executive Director

December, 1973   National Acupuncture Research Society

CHAPTER 1

History of the Development of Ear Acupuncture

Chairman Mao once said: "Traditional Chinese medicine is a great treasure house which ought to be explored and further enriched." Ear acupuncture is just one component of this treasure, representing the accumulated experiences of the laboring Chinese people in using the needling method for the conquest of diseases. Our endeavor to trace the historical development of acupuncture will not only illustrate the acupuncture theory but also enable us to explore and organize the great heritage of traditional Chinese medicine.

In *The Yellow Emperor's Classic of Internal Medicine (Nei ching)*, the first medical work published as early as 400-200 B.C., the ear is considered not as an isolated organ but intimately connected with all organs of the body, five viscera,[1] and six bowels.[2] In the chapter "Mystical Gate *(Ling shu):* Treatise on the Bad Spirit and the Diseases of Internal Organs," it is pointed out, "There are twelve meridians and 365 branch vessels for the circulation of blood and air. Blood and air circulate upwards to the face

---

[1] Five viscera *(wu-tsang)* are liver, heart, spleen, lungs, and kidneys.

[2] Six bowels *(liu-fu)* are bile, small intestine, stomach, large intestine, gallbladder, and *san-chiao*, or triple warmer, which was previously considered an imaginary organ but is now identified as a combination of internal organs composed of three sections, one at the cardiac end of the stomach, another within the stomach, and a third around the ureters.

and orifices . . . and peripheral blood and air circulate to the ear to facilitate the power of hearing." In other words, blood and air circulate through twelve meridians and their 365 accessory points to infiltrate the five sense organs, seven orifices, and brain marrow . . . and peripheral blood and air circulate through branch vessels to the ear to facilitate the power of hearing. This generally sums up the relationship between ear and the vascular system. More explicit knowledge is contained in the several chapters of *The Yellow Emperor's Classic of Internal Medicine* and has been enriched by physicians of succeeding dynasties.

According to "Mystical Gate: Treatise on Meridians and Vessels," "the meridian of the Lesser *Yang*[3] of the hand extends upwards to the back of the ear, enters the upper corner of the ear, and from the back of the ear enters the center of the ear, and then passes the front of the ear." Again, "The meridian of the Great *Yang* of the hand reaches the center of the ear." "The meridian of the Sunlight *(Yang-ming)* of the foot extends to the front of the ear." "The meridian of the Lesser *Yang* of the foot reaches the back of the ear, enters the center of the ear, and passes the front of the ear." "The meridian of the Great *Yang* of the foot extends to the upper corner of the ear." "The branch vessel of the Sunlight meridian of the hand reaches the ear and joins with the main vessel." These passages show that the circulation system of the six *Yang* of the twelve meridians passes through the ear.

Although the six *Yin* meridians do not directly pass through the ear, according to the differentiation of twelve meridians in "Mystical Gate: Vessel Classification," their circulation routes remain the same, that is, the *Yin* meridians join with their corresponding *Yang* meridians, and each of the *Yang* meridians finally rejoins with its corresponding *Yin* meridian. Therefore, through the system of transmitting and receiving, the six *Yin* meridians are also indirectly connected with the ear.

It is also pointed out in "Plain Dialogue *(Su-wen)*: Treatise on

---

3 *Yang* means, literally, "the sunny side of a hill" and *yin* "the shady side of a hill." *Yin* and *yang* are considered the primogenial elements from which the universe was evolved. When applied to the human body, the balance of *yin* and *yang* means harmony or health.

Acupuncture," "The meridians of both the Lesser *Yin* and Great *Yin* of the hand and foot, and the Sunlight meridian of the foot are five meridians converging in the ear." This supplements the content of "Mystical Gate: Treatise on Meridians and Vessels."

In *The Study of Eight Special Meridians (Chi-ching pai-mai kao)* published in 1572 during the Ming period, the relationship between meridians and the ear is further expounded on the basis of the study of eight special meridians. The two *Yin* and *Yang* exciters *(chiao-mai)* control the *Yin* and *Yang* meridians of the left and right side and extend upwards to the rear of the ears. The *Yang* keeper *(Wei-mai)*, a network connecting all the *Yang* meridians, also passes through the head to reach the ear. Therefore, according to "Mystical Gate: Oral Inquiry," "The ear is the converging place of the main vessels," that is to say, many meridians and vessels are joined in the ear. All these treatises show that the relationship between ear and meridians and vessels is considerably complicated.

Materials concerning the relationship between ear and internal organs are abundant in the medical literature of ancient times. It is recorded in "Mystical Gate: Pulse Measurement" that "Air from the kidney is connected with the ear; thus when there is harmony in the kidneys the ears can distinguish the five musical notes." In "Plain Dialogue: Treatise on the Truth of the Golden Chamber," it is said: "The orifice of the heart is the ear." The physiological relationship between the ear on the one hand and the heart and kidney on the other is thus made clear.

In "Plain Dialogue: Treatise on the Harmony of Internal Organs," it is recorded: "When spleen is in disorder all nine orifices are obstructed." In "Plain Dialogue: A General Discourse on the Fullness and the Insufficiency (of the body)," it is also said: "That the head aches, the ears hear sound, and the nine orifices do not function properly is caused by the malfunction of the stomach and intestines." These passages explain the intimate physiological and pathological relations between the ear on the one hand and the spleen, stomach, and large and small intestines of the digestive system on the other.

In "Plain Dialogue: Treatise on Seasons as Patterns of the

Viscera," it is pointed out that "Sickness of liver . . . when it is insufficient the ear cannot hear . . . when air circulates backwards, it causes headaches and deafness, loss of acute perception." This account suggests the mutual pathological relationship between ear and liver. Finally, in "Mystical Gate: Treatise on the Sea of Marrow," it is said that "When the sea of marrow is insufficient it causes head spin and ear buzz." Here the sea of marrow refers to brain tissue. It is clear that ancients millennia ago recognized the connection between ear and brain tissue.

The relationship between lung, one of the five viscera, and ear is recorded in *Difficult Classic*.[4] "The Fortieth Difficult Passage" says the "Lung controls hearing . . . and directs ear to hear sound." This expounds the relationship between lung and ear. In *Criteria in Diagnosis and Treatment*[5] published in 1602 during the Ming period, it is suggested that "When air in the lungs is insufficient . . . the ear turns deaf." The relationship between ear and lung is thus explained on the basis of pathological phenomena. In *Illustrations of Miscellaneous Diseases (Tsa ping yuan-liu hsi-chu)* published in 1773 during the Ch'ing period, it is more explicitly stated, "Lung controls air . . . which spreads all over the body to converge in the ear." These treatises form the theoretical basis of the relationship between ear and five viscera and six bowels.

The above records found in Chinese medical literature fully show that our ancestors long ago recognized the intimate relationship between ear and vessels and internal organs. According to traditional Chinese medicine, meridians and vessels, spreading all over the body, are transmitting routes for air and blood. The ear is connected to every part of the body because of the ceaseless circulation of air and blood through these meridians and vessels. The outer and branch vessels serve the function of connecting with the outer limbs to form the harmonious relationship between the ear, four limbs, and a hundred bones. The inward circulation

---

[4] *Difficult Classic (Nan ching)*, in 2 volumes, was written by Pien Ch'iao of the Chou dynasty (1122-255 B.C.). It contains explanations and annotations of 81 difficult passages selected from *The Yellow Emperor's Classic of Internal Medicine*.
  [5] *Criteria of Diagnosis and Treatment (Cheng-chih chun-sheng)*, a stupendous 120 volumes, was authored by Wang-Ken-tang.

system of meridians and vessels through the internal organs furthers the intimate relationship and mutual influence between the ear, five viscera, and six bowels. Thus in *A Treasury of Health (wei-sheng pao-chien)* published in 1281 during the Yuan period, it is pointed out: "Five viscera, six bowels, and twelve meridians are joined in the ear." This clearly explains that the ear joins with the body to form the unified, inseparable whole, a theory which forms the basis for diagnosis and treatment in the posterior.

The examination of the outer ear for diagnosis is also recorded in *The Yellow Emperor's Classic of Internal Medicine.* In "Mystical Gate: Teaching of the Master" can be found the record of "detecting good or bad conditions of the ear" for diagnosing kidneys. *The Classic of Central Organs*[6] also records ear examination as a means of predicting ailments and recovery. It is thus clear that ear examination as a means for diagnosis has a history of almost 2,000 years.

Records concerning ear treatment for curing diseases can be traced back to the period of the Warring States. Ko Hung (281-341), in his *Prescriptions for Emergencies (Chou-hou pei-chi fang)*, a renowned work of the Tsin period, quotes Ch'in Yueh-jen's[7] (born circa 5th century B.C.) treatment of death by suffocation, "using a pipe to blow into the left ear three times and then the right ear three times." It also records the experience of the Han physician Chang Chung-ching (born 2nd-3rd century A.D.). "For treatment of sudden death with eyes closed, pour leek juice into ear." These records show that the ancients attempted treatment of diseases through the ear. Later in the early years of the T'ang period, Sun Szu-mo (581-682) in his *Thousand Gold Remedies (Chien chin fang)* reported many cases of using the ear for treating diseases. For instance, "Jaundice and a variety of epidemics common in winter and summer can be cured by applying acupuncture and moxibustion to the upper ridge in the center of the ear." Again,

---

6 *The Classic of Central Organs (Chung tsang ching)* is often erroneously attributed to Hua T'o of the period of the Three Kingdoms. It was actually published in the Sung period of unknown authorship.

7 Ch'in Yueh-jen, better known as Pien Ch'iao, was the author of *Difficult Classic* (see Note 4) and perhaps the most famous of ancient physicians.

"deafness and buzzing in the ear" can be cured by applying moxibustion to the vessel of the *Yang* keeper.

In *The Prescription of Treating Malaria (Chih yeh fang)* by Ch'en Ts'ang-ch'i (born circa 730's), published in the middle of the T'ang period, it is said that malaria can be cured by filling up both ears with bolted snake skin. In *A Treasury of Health*, mentioned earlier, "convulsions in children" is said to be curable by applying moxibustion to the blue vein behind the ear. In *The Compendium of Acupuncture and Moxibustion (Chen chiu ta-ch'eng)*, published in 1602 during the Ming period, it is recorded that cataract can be cured by applying moxibustion to the ear summit point. The book also contains a section of the historical development in the application of acupuncture and moxibustion to various points of the ear. Furthermore, many methods in curing ailments by treating the ear are widely used in China's countryside, such as needling the ear lobe for curing pinkeye, pricking the vein behind the ear to release blood for curing eye infection, and needling the periphery of the outer ear for curing pain in the ribs and diarrhea. The method of ear massage as one of the techniques of remedial massages shows that using two hands to pull ear lobes can cure headache and using fingers to rub ear lobes can cure convulsions in children. Both methods are effective. It is thus obvious that China has a long history of applying acupuncture and moxibustion to the ear for curing diseases.

There were new developments in recent years. In 1956, the Health Department of Laisi county of Shantung province first reported that ear acupuncture could cure throat numbness. In 1957, the French physician P. Nogier made a careful study of the connection between the ear and other parts of the body based on his knowledge of acupuncture and moxibustion. He applied his research result to clinical treatment, added many ear acupuncture points, and thus contributed to the development of ear acupuncture.

In 1958, encouraged by the Party's General Line in Socialist reconstruction, the knowledge of acupuncture and moxibustion was greatly expanded. There was a massive movement to study and apply ear acupuncture across the nation. As a result, general conclusions were drawn from several hundred clinical cases, the scope of ear acupuncture was greatly enlarged, and the knowledge of ear acupuncture greatly enriched. However, people like Liu Shao-ch'i[8] did everything they could to promote the revisionist line in medicine and health. They spread erroneous ideas such as "Chinese medicine is unscientific" and "insertion of the needle can only kill pain but cannot cure disease" that seriously hampered the exploration ond systematization of ear acupuncture and rendered it to the state of oblivion. Since the Cultural Revolution dispelled the erroneous ideas of Liu Shao-ch'i and his associates, ear acupuncture has been again broadly applied all over the country and reached a new landmark as a result of the joint efforts of the masses, physicians and health personnel. At present the number of ear acupuncture points has been increased to over 200. These acupuncture points and their clinical application reflect to a certain extent both traditional Chinese medical theory and anatomy in modern medical science and provide rich experience for combining Chinese and Western medical knowledge for treatment of diseases.

In recent years advanced research has been carried on for diagnosis based on pain felt at the sensitive point when pressed, bloodshot spot, discoloration, papules, small blisters, skin peeling, skin erosion, and the increase of bioelectric conductivity of the skin of the outer ear. The methods of stimulating ear acupuncture points are also increased to more than a dozen—from simple needling to leaving the needle in place, electric needling, applying ointment, injecting medicine, blocking the acupuncture point, wet needling, warm needling, pricking with the needle, blood letting, moxibustion, ear squeezing, pumping in air, ear massage, and rubbing with fingers. The scope of application is continually enlarged and the efficacy of treatment continually improved. Finally, the development of ear acupuncture anesthesia opens a new

---

8 Liu Shao-ch'i, formerly chairman of the People's Republic of China, was accused of revisionism during the Cultural Revolution.

dimension in this traditional Chinese medical treatment.

The social imperialist[9], however, has used all kinds of rumors and slanders to belittle ear acupuncture and even maliciously attacked it in some periodicals. This type of ugly distortion only exposes the ignorance of the social imperialist in medical science and their reactionary nature in politics.

In the process of studying and applying ear acupuncture we profoundly felt that the human body is always in a state of unity of opposites in which all parts maintain intimate relationship, competing with each other, depending on each other, connected with each other, and restraining each other. Any pathological development in one part of the body can affect the whole body or other organs; the condition of the whole body in turn can affect the pathological development in a certain part. No disease exists in isolation but affects and is affected by some other factors. The method of ear acupuncture is based on this fundamental principle of unity of opposites. Human being is regarded as a unified, continually moving entity and the development of disease in the human body, the result of struggle between contradictions. Chairman Mao's brilliant philosophical ideas are the powerful ideological weapon in our learning and developing ear acupuncture. By applying Chairman Mao's brilliant philosophical ideas, we combined the revolutionary spirit of daring to think and daring to do with the scientific method of experimentation in the exploration and application of ear acupuncture. Through synthesis, analysis, and discussion, we repeatedly adjust, locate, and determine the general pathological inter-reacting principle between ear and internal organs, body surface, and four limbs, further our systematic understanding of ear acupuncture points, enrich and develop the significance and content of many acupuncture points, and thus acquire better treatment results.

In the last few years we went through several hundred thousand treatments, cured more than 200 varieties of diseases in which the results for 150 were excellent and many were common diseases, recurring diseases, and some chronic diseases of organic

---

9 That is, the Soviet Union.

origin. The extensive clinical application of ear acupuncture in recent years shows that this simple method has multiple uses, attains speedy results, demonstrates efficacy, and is inexpensive. It enriches the treasure house of traditional Chinese medicine, and at the same time its scientific principle is a powerful repudiation of bourgeois metaphysical philosophy.

"The history of mankind is a history of continual development from the kingdom of necessity to the kingdom of freedom." There is no end to the development of knowledge, nor is there end to the development from no freedom to freedom. Ear acupuncture is still in the process of development with many problems yet to be answered. Let us move forward, under the direction of Chairman Mao's revolutionary line, to continually explore and organize Chinese medical heritage and to strive for the creation of a unified, new medical science in China.

CHAPTER 2

Merits of Ear Acupuncture Treatment

For the past ten years in the development of ear acupuncture treatment, we came to realize many merits of this method, including its broad application, quick and effective results, easy manipulation of the needle, fast mastery of the skills, practical and inexpensive, convenient to the patient, and with little side effect. In the past few years we learned to apply ear acupuncture to diagnosis, prevention of illness, and anaesthesia. The broad clinical application of ear acupuncture reflects Chairman Mao's great strategic policy "Be prepared against war, be prepared against natural disasters, and do everything for the people." It helps promote revolution, promote production, promote construction, and promote national defense. It accelerates the development and consolidation of the system of cooperative medical care in the countryside.

Application to a Broad Variety of Diseases

In our attempt to use ear acupuncture for the service of workers, peasants, and soldiers, we cured not only functional diseases but also chronic, inveterate organic diseases. These include functional bleeding of the uterus, appendicitis, inner ear dizziness (Ménière's syndrome), neurogenic dermatitis, dermatophiliasis, allergic rhinitis, intestinal disorder, impotence, pulse-

lessness (arteritis), obstructive vasculitis, disorder of internal secretion, sequela of brain trauma, dwarfism, mumps, and inflammation of the middle ear (otitis media).

Quick and Effective Results

All the diseases which can be treated by ear acupuncture can
be quickly and effectively put under control. For example:

(1) Quick to kill pain: External wounds, postoperative pains, and
pains caused by inflammations in cases such as sprain, injury from
crush, strain, disjoint, bone fracture, chronic ulcer, intestinal
cramps, puerperal uteralgia, renal stones (urinary lithiasis), ascaris
(roundworm) infection in the gall, can all be stopped in a matter
of a few minutes.

(2) Quick to reduce inflammation: Before all kinds of inflammation suppurate, ear acupuncture can control and reduce inflammation within several to twenty-four hours after the insertion of
the needle. Especially in cases such as barley grain (hordeolum or
stye), chalazion, carbuncles, mumps, frostbite, bronchitis, pneu-
monia, tonsillitis, acute conjunctivitis, appendicitis, enteritis, and
diarrhea.

(3) Quick to stop itching: Itching caused by dermatophiliasis,
contact dermatitis, and prickly heat can be halted and cured by
inserting the needle.

(4) Emergency treatment: Cases of emergency such as shock,
heat stroke, and convulsion can be controlled in several minutes
to a few hours after the insertion of the needle to facilitate the
return to normal blood pressure.

(5) Quick for reducing fever: Generally, high and persistent
fever can be lowered by needling to release blood. Sometimes the
body temperature will be reduced or return to normal half an hour
after needling.

Easy Manipulation of the Needle

The application of ear acupuncture does not require special
facilities, nor is it restricted by location and weather condition.

Whether indoors, outdoors, in open field, factory workshop, battle-field, trenches, or classroom, ear acupuncture can be applied. When no acupuncture needle is available, regular needle or pin will do. If necessary using a matchstick to press on the sensitive point can cure headache, strain, pleuroneuralgia, and stomachache.

Easy Mastery of the Skills

Ear acupuncture treatment is the insertion of a needle in the outer ear where acupuncture points are concentrated. Not too many of them are commonly used, and their locations fall into a definite pattern. Many of the acupuncture points, named according to the corresponding anatomical parts, are therefore easy to learn and easy to remember. As a result, most people with some medical knowledge can learn ear acupuncture in a matter of several hours. Thus, ear acupuncture has acquired great popularity among the Chinese people. In our army unit some commanders learned the ear acupuncture method for the treatment of some common dis-eases within a short time. Some patients, after being treated for a certain time, not only were cured but also learned the ear acu-puncture method to treat others with good results.

Economy and Convenience

The use of ear acupuncture takes only a few acupuncture needles, some sterilized cotton balls, and a bottle of alcohol. Patients welcome ear acupuncture because it cures ailments with no cost or cures serious diseases with little cost. It is convenient for diagnosis and treatment. It does not affect the patient's job in the process of treatment. If a patient is too busy to undergo treat-ment, he can simply have the needle left in place to save extra trips to the clinic.

Little or No Side Effect

In our experiences of inserting the experimental needle in ourselves and of treating patients, we come to the conclusion that except for some peculiar sensation felt when the needle is being inserted, there is no other side effect. Sometimes, when the needle is inserted too deeply into the sympathetic (*chiao-kan hsueh*), a sense of heaviness can be felt at the temples. When the needle is inserted into acupuncture points such as the suprarenal gland, internal secretion, heart, and kidney, sometimes the patient may suffer from a dizzy spell, fainting, heart palpitating, vomiting, lower limb chillness, or body numbness. Such reactions may be reduced or disappear the moment the needle is withdrawn slightly. Occasionally, patients are found to suffer needle sickness. In that case, they only have to lie flat for a couple of minutes to recover. If the needles and the outer ear are not fully sterilized, ear infection or ear shriveling may develop. Both can be easily avoided with sufficient precaution.

Diagnosis and Differential Diagnosis

In recent years there has been rapid development in ear acupuncture, and a good deal of new knowledge has been acquired. (For explicit methods, see chapters on "Diagnosis by Examining the Auricle" and "A Brief Discussion of Ear Acupuncture Points Locating Devices and Their Application.") It has reference value for differential diagnosis of atypical acute abdominal diseases such as ovarian cyst, renal stone (urinary lithiasis), appendicitis, and gallstone.

Prevention of Diseases

In the last few years we obtained satisfactory results in the preventive treatment of mumps, epidemic influenza, and malaria. For comparative experiment, two companies were selected in the prevention of malaria. In one company, ear acupuncture was applied every ten days by inserting the needle at five acupuncture points—suprarenal gland, internal secretion, dermis, spleen, and liver. After a total of twelve treatments, the annual malaria rate in this company was 1.2%. In another company no preventive measures were taken, and the annual malaria rate was as high as

8.5%. We also discovered that of those who had been treated by ear acupuncture, 80% showed an increase in appetite, improvement in sleep, and strengthening in resistance. They rarely caught cold or suffered influenza.

Acupuncture Anaesthesia

The use of ear acupuncture anaesthesia was rapidly developed in the last few years. It allows surgical operation to proceed while the patient remains fully conscious. The advantage is that the patient's body is able to function fully in the process of operation and his will to recover is also strengthened. For those physically weak patients who cannot withstand drug anaesthesia before operation, ear acupuncture anaesthesia is much safer and subsequent recovery much faster. It is a good way to carry out Chairman Mao's instructions "Be prepared against war, be prepared against natural disasters, and do everything for the people." At present, ear acupuncture anesthesia is used not only in removing tonsils and teeth and in treating disjoints but also in operations of chest, abdomen, four limbs, ear, nose, throat, and eye. It is conceivable that its application will be increasingly broadened.

Ear acupuncture treatment is a new development in the medical and therapeutic field but although it has many merits, it also has limitations. For some diseases, its curing efficacy is not lasting or is only relieving, such as in cases like emphysema, epilepsy, and chronic pains in the loins and legs. Therefore, treating ear acupuncture as a panacea is contrary to the dialectic theory. Inserting the needle in the outer ear often produces a special sensation which, especially in continual treatment, may more or less have a negative effect on the patient's active cooperation. In the clinical application of ear acupuncture, aside from making best use of its merits, sometimes complementary use of body acupuncture, Chinese herbal medicine, and modern medicine for reinforcing its curing efficacy can also be considered.

CHAPTER 3

The Structure and Organization
of the Auricle

The auricle (outer ear) consists of complex-shaped elastic cartilage, a small amount of fat, and connective tissue. It is covered with skin underneath which spread rich nerves, blood vessels, and lymph glands. The front surface is concave and the back surface correspondingly convex. The upper 3/4 to 4/5 of the auricle is primarily formed of elastic cartilage, while the lower 1/4 to 1/5, or the lobule, consists of fat and connective tissue. The skin of the concave side is more tightly attached to the cartilage.

Anatomical Features of the Auricle (Plate 1)

(1) helix: the inverted rim of the auricle.

(2) crus of helix: the prominent oblique ridge in the depression, an extension of the helix.

(3) auricular tubercle: the slight projection in the free margin of the helix.

(4) anthelix: a prominent semicircular ridge lying opposite to the helix.

(5) upper crura of anthelix: the upper ridge of the superiorly divided anthelix.

15

(6) lower crura of anthelix: the lower ridge of the divided anthelix.

(7) triangular fossa: the triangular depression formed by the upper and lower ridges of the anthelix.

(8) scaphoid fossa: the trough-shaped depression between the helix and the anthelix.

(9) tragus: the petal-shaped projection over the entrance to the meatus, sometimes called auricular pearl.

(10) anterior incisure: the depression separating the tragus from the crus of the helix.

(11) antitragus: the projection lying opposite to the tragus and at the lower end of the anthelix.

(12) intertragic incisure: the deep notch between the tragus and the antitragus.

(13) lobule: the skin-formed, flattened, rounded lobe at the lower part of the auricle.

(14) cymba concha: the superior part of the concavity above the crus of helix.

(15) cavum concha: the inferior part of the concavity below the crus of helix.

(16) external acoustic meatus: the auditory canal situated in the cavum concha and shielded by the tragus.

(17) posterior auricular sulcus: the notch between the anthelix and the antitragus.

(18) tail of helix: the inferior cartilageless rim of the helix.

Distribution of Nerves in the Auricle

The nerves distributed in the auricle are extremely rich; they are derived from the trigeminal nerve, facial nerve, glossopharyngeal nerve, vagus nerve, major auricular nerve, and minor occipital nerve. Their distribution is as follows:

The Auricular Branch of the Auriculotemporal Nerve: The auriculotemporal nerve, derived from the trigeminal nerve, has 3-4 minor branches distributed at the helix and the anterior of the triangular fossa, lower crura of anthelix, upper anterior of the crus of helix, cymba concha, tragus, and lobule.

The Auricular Branch of the Vagus Nerve: It is derived from the jugular vein ganglion of the vagus nerve, then courses anteriorly, and merges with the facial nerve in the facial canal. When the facial nerve passes the mastoid air cells, it departs from the facial canal, extends upward along the posterior of the auricle, and divides into two branches at the lower half of the trough, called anterior branches of the vagus nerve, which penetrate the elastic cartilage to spread all over the cavum concha and the external acoustic meatus.

The Auricular Branch of the Facial Nerve: It is derived from the facial nerve and emerges after the facial canal passes the mastoid air cells. It extends upward along the posterior trough and splits into the posterior branch which spreads at the posterior of the auricle and the anterior branch which penetrates the elastic cartilage to spread in the cymba concha, lower part of the crus of helix, and middle part of the crura of anthelix. Its ends can reach as far as the lower part of the triangular fossa.

There is a connective branch of the glossopharyngeal nerve and the vagus nerve, that is, the auricular branch of the vagus nerve contains the fibre of the glossopharyngeal nerve and its area of distribution may correspond with that of the vagus nerve. The auricular branch of the vagus nerve courses over a certain distance inside the facial canal, and thus it is impossible to separate mixed fibres in the vagus nerve and the facial nerve and furthermore, it is possible that there is the common distribution of the vagus nerve and the facial nerve in the conchae. Their precise distribution is yet to be explored.

The Major Auricular Nerve: It is derived from the cervical plexus and courses superficially along the sternocleidomastoideus muscle. It splits at the upper part of the lobule into the anterior and posterior branches. The anterior branch passes through the lobule to the front (depressed area) and then splits in two. The larger one courses along the scaphoid fossa to spread all over the lower 2/3 of the scaphoid fossa, anthelix, triangular fossa, cymba concha, and part of the crus of the helix; the other branch spreads over the middle upper part of the scaphoid fossa and the middle of the helix. It also reaches the lobule below the intertragic incisure. The posterior branch spreads over the middle of the auricle.

The minor occipital nerve also comes from the cervical plexus and courses upward along the back rim of the sternocleidomastoideus muscle with branches spreading over the upper part of the auricle. Its posterior branch spreads over the upper 1/3 of the posterior of the auricle. Its anterior branch and connective branch spread over the upper part of the helix and the scaphoid fossa, upper crura of the anthelix, and part of the triangular fossa. The major occipital nerve and the minor occipital nerve partially join up, and thus the fibres of the former may spread through the latter to the auricle.

It is clear from the above description of the nerve distribution that the origins of the nerves in the several areas of the auricle are different; major part of the helix, anthelix, and scaphoid fossa is covered with the major auricular nerve, while only a small upper part of the same area is covered with the minor auricular nerve.

The nerves in the triangular fossa come from the auriculotemporal nerve, major auricular nerve, and minor occipital nerve, and form a nerve plexus.

The nerves in the cymba concha and cavum concha include, in addition to a few branches of the major auricular nerve, primarily branches of the facial nerve, vagus nerve, and trigeminal nerve. All these nerves join together here to form a nerve plexus.

The nerves in the lobule come from the auriculotemporal nerve and the major auricular nerve.

The upper 1/3 of the posterior of the auricle is covered by the minor occipital nerve and its lower 2/3 by the major auricular nerve and the posterior branch of the facial nerve. Furthermore, the auricular branch of the vagus nerve also spreads over the depressed area at the posterior of the auricle.

The nerves in the derma layer of the auricle form a denser nerve net. The nerve fibres from the nerve net form the tips of sensory nerves in the epidermis, around the hair follicles, and in the dermis. There is also a minor nerve plexus accompanying blood vessels to enter the elastic cartilage to form the tips of the sensory nerves.

Distribution of Blood Vessels in the Auricle

There is plenty of blood supply in the auricle, primarily from the superficial temporal artery of the external carotid artery and the posterior auricular artery.

Three to four anterior auricular branches of the superficial temporal artery nourish the area covered by the anterior branch of the auriculotemporal nerves. The posterior and anterior branches are derived from the posterior auricular artery. The posterior branch together with the facial nerve and the posterior branch of the major auricular nerve spreads over and nourishes the posterior of the auricle. The anterior branch of the superficial temporal artery, along with the anterior branch of the major auricular nerve, passes the lobule to reach the anterior of the auricle and nourishes the area covered by the major auricle nerve (Plates 10–12).

The veins in the anterior of the auricle are minute and many are directly linked with the superficial temporal vein. The 3-5 veins at the posterior of the auricle extend along the auricular rim to the side of the head and join with the posterior auricular veins.

Lymphatics of the Auricle

The auricle is full of lymphatics in net-like shape. The lymphatics of the anterior auricle drain into the parotid lymph nodes. The lymphatics of the posterior auricle generally drain into the posterior auricular lymph nodes.

The above description provides for some basic knowledge about the auricle morphology for exploring and studying the function of the auricle in clinical diagnosis and treatment. A complete understanding of the structure and organization of the auricle, especially of the circulating routes of the arteries and veins, still requires further scientific experiment and research.

CHAPTER 4

The Distribution and Location of Ear Acupuncture Points

Ear acupuncture points are those auricular points which show the *yang* (positive) reaction when viscera, bowels, limbs, and external organs suffer ailments. Inserting the needle at a particular point may cure a particular ailment. This point is called ear acupuncture point.

A *yang* reaction point means that a particular auricular point may produce a series of reactions, such as discoloration, erupting rash, skin peeling, deformation, feeling pain when pressed, and reduction in electric resistance. Thus, the ear acupuncture point is also called reaction point, sensitive point, pain point, or high conductivity point.

After repeated experiment and research by medical personnel all over China and the medical team in our unit, we have identified more than 200 ear acupuncture points. The distribution of the commonly used ear acupuncture points at the auricle is as shown in Table 4-1 and Plates 2 through 8:

TABLE 4-1

The Anatomical Locations of Ear Acupuncture Points

	Ear Acupuncture Point	Anatomical Location	Remarks
Lobule	lower palate	at the inner ⅓ of the upper line of zone 2.	The lobule is corresponding to the cheek. Draw a horizontal line from the intertragic incisure as a dividing line and then draw two parallel lines to divide the lobule into three equal parts. Divide the top-most horizontal line into three equal parts and draw two vertical lines to divide the lobule into 9 zones.
	upper palate	at the lower ¼ of the outer line in zone 2.	
	tongue	between lower and upper palate, leaning slightly upward.	
	upper jowl	center of zone 3.	
	lower jowl	middle of the upper line in zone 3.	
	eye	center of zone 5.	
	inner ear	slightly above the center of zone 6.	
	tonsil	center of zone 8.	
	cheek area	surrounding the line dividing zones 5 and 6.	
	tooth extraction anaesthesia point	two points at the outer-lower corners of zones 1 and 4 respectively.	
Antitragus	parotid gland	the highest point in the middle zone.	The arc-shaped antitragus, corresponding to the head, is divided into three zones. For the convenience of description, the outer upper area is called the upper zone and the inner lower area the lower zone.
	asthma	0.2 cm. anteriorly lower than parotid gland.	
	testicle	0.2 cm. posteriorly lower than parotid gland.	
	brain point	the highest point at the center of the upper zone.	
	occiput	on the rim of the cartilage of the antitragus, opposite brain point in the upper zone.	
	forehead	on the rim of the cartilage of the antitragus, center of the lower zone.	
	temple	on the rim of the cartilage of the antitragus between occiput and forehead.	

TABLE 4-1 (cont'd)

	Ear Acupuncture Point	Anatomical Location	Remarks
Antitragus	apex	about 0.15 cm. below occiput.	
	lower dermis	at the inner side of the lower zone.	
	excitement point	at the middle between testicle and lung point.	
Scaphoid Fossa	collar bone	at the bottom of the scaphoid fossa on the same level as heart.	scaphoid fossa corresponds to the upper limbs.
	finger	at the lower rim of the helix in upper scaphoid fossa. Divide the area between collar bone and finger into four equal zones.	
	shoulder joint	in the first zone above collar bone.	
	shoulder	in the second zone above collar bone.	
	elbow	in the third zone above collar bone.	
	wrist	in the fourth zone above collar bone.	
	nephritis point	at the lower-outer side of collar bone.	
	appendix point	altogether three points: one slightly above finger, another above shoulder, and a third below collarbone.	
	urticaria point	between finger and wrist.	
Anthelix	vertebra of neck	at the initial rising point of the anthelix.	The anthelix corresponds to the vertebra.
	sacral vertebra	at the initial rising point of the upper and lower crura of anthelix. Divide the area between vertebra of neck and sacral vertebra into 2 equal zones.	
	thoracic vertebra	in the first zone above vertebra of neck.	

TABLE 4-1 (cont'd)

Ear Acupuncture Point	Anatomical Location	Remarks
Anthelix		
lumbar vertebra	in the second zone above vertebra of neck; another vertebra area at the inner rim of the anthelix.	
neck	between vertebra of neck and thoracic vertebra, leaning inward.	
thorax	between thoracic vertebra and lumbar vertebra, leaning inward.	
abdomen	between lumbar vertebra and sacral vertebra, leaning inward.	
outer abdomen	on the outer side of the anthelix, roughly on the same level as kidney.	
heat point	between sacral vertebra and lumbago point, roughly on the same level as buttock.	
thyroid gland	above and outside vertebra of neck, parallel to neck.	
mammary gland	above thoracic vertebra; two points forming an equilateral triangle with thoracic vertebra.	
appendix-abdomen point	on the outer rim of the anthelix, parallel to kidney.	
lumbago point	0.2 cm. below sacral vertebra.	
Upper Crura of Anthelix		
toe	at the end of upper crura of anthelix, leaning outward.	The upper crura of anthelix corresponds to the lower limbs.
heel	at the end of upper crura of anthelix, leaning inward.	
ankle joint	below toe and heel, forming a triangle with the two points.	
knee	at the departing section of upper crura of anthelix, above and outside sacral vertebra.	

TABLE 4-1 (cont'd)

	Ear Acupuncture Point	Anatomical Location	Remarks
Upper Crura of Anthelix	hip joint	midway between sacral vertebra and toe.	
	knee joint	midway between hip joint and toe.	
Lower Crura of Anthelix	buttock	at the inner rim of the departing section of lower crura of anthelix.	The lower crura of anthelix corresponds to the buttocks.
	sympathetic	at the end of lower crura of anthelix.	
	sciatic nerve	midway between buttock and sympathetic.	
Triangular Fossa	uterus	the lowest point of the depression in the triangular fossa.	
	shen-men	near the end ½ - ⅓ of upper crura of anthelix.	
	pelvis cavum	at the cross point of upper and lower crura of anthelix.	
	lowering pressure point	at the end of upper crura of anthelix.	
	asthma point	about 0.2 cm. outside uterus.	
	thigh joint	at the upper rim of lower crura of anthelix, forming a triangle with sciatic and buttock.	
	constipation point	near the center section of lower crura of anthelix, above and inside sciatic, on a horizontal level.	
	hepatitis point	midway between asthma point and *shen-men*.	

TABLE 4-1 (cont'd)

Ear Acupuncture Point	Anatomical Location	Remarks
mouth	below crus of helix, above and outside external acoustic meatus.	The peripheral area of crus of helix corresponds to digestive system.
stomach	at the diminishing point of crus of helix.	
oesophagus	at the lower rim of crus of helix, about ⅓ left of the center between mouth and stomach.	
cardia	below the lower rim of crus of helix, about ⅓ right of the center between mouth and stomach.	
duodenum	at the upper rim of crus of helix, opposite cardia.	
small intestine	at the upper rim of crus of helix, opposite oesophagus.	
large intestine	at the upper rim of crus of helix, opposite mouth.	
appendix	between large and small intestines.	
diaphragm	at crus of helix, forming a right angle with mouth and oesophagus.	The crus of helix corresponds to diaphragm.
ear center	outside diaphragm, forming a vertical line with oesophagus and cardia.	
bladder	below lower crura of anthelix and above large intestine.	The cymba concha corresponds to abdomen.
kidney	below lower crura of anthelix and pelvis cavum.	
ureter	between bladder and kidney.	
prostate	inside of bladder, below sympathetic.	
liver	at the rear and above stomach.	
pancreas gall	between liver and kidney.	

Peripheral Area of Crus of Helix

Crus of Helix

Cymba Concha

TABLE 4-1 (cont'd)

Ear Acupuncture Point	Anatomical Location	Remarks
Cymba Concha		
pancreatitis point	at the lower ⅔ between duodenum and pancreas gall.	
ascites point	at the center of kidney, pancreas gall and small intestine.	
drunk point	at the top ⅓ between kidney and small intestine.	
Cavum Concha		
heart	at the lowest point of the depression of cavum concha, showing reflection.	The cavum concha corresponds to thorax.
spleen	below and outside stomach.	
lung	above and below heart.	
bronchus	in the lung area, about ⅓ from the inner border.	
tubercle point	at the center of the lung area.	
bronchiectasia	at ⅓ from the outer border of the lung area.	
trachea	at external acoustic meatus, parallel to heart.	
cirrhosis area	in a line at the middle of hepatomegalia area.	
hepatomegalia area	at the diminishing point of crus of helix, an area located outside stomach.	
triple warmer	at the center of three points —inner nose, internal secretion, and lung.	
hepatitis area	between stomach and spleen at a slightly lower level.	
new eye point	at the center of three points —oesophagus, cardia, and lung.	

TABLE 4-1 (cont'd)

	Ear Acupuncture Point	Anatomical Location	Remarks
Tragus	inner nose	at the inside lower ½ of tragus.	The tragus corresponds to nose and throat.
	throat	at the inside upper ½ of tragus.	
	suprarenal gland	at the lower ½ of tragus.	
	tragus apex	at the upper ½ of tragus.	
	outer nose	at the front rim of tragus cartilage, forming a triangle with tragus apex and suprarenal gland.	
	thirst point	midway between tragus apex and outer nose but at a slightly upper level.	
	hunger point	midway between suprarenal gland and outer nose but at a slightly lower level.	
	high blood pressure point	midway between suprarenal gland and eye$_1$.	
	nose-ear purity	midway between tragus apex and suprarenal gland, at the rim of tragus cartilage.	
Intertragic Incisure	internal secretion	at 0.2 cm. inside intertragic incisure.	The intertragic incisure corresponds to internal secretion.
	ovary	below dermis at the front side.	
	eye$_1$	at the front lower side of intertragic incisure.	
	eye$_2$	at the rear lower side of intertragic incisure.	
	rising pressure point	between eye$_1$ and eye$_2$.	
Anterior Incisure	outer ear	at the front depression of anterior incisure.	The anterior incisure corresponds to outer ear.
	cardiac point	at the depression above tragus apex.	

TABLE 4-1 (cont'd)

Ear Acupuncture Point	Anatomical Location	Remarks
Posterior Auricular Sulcus		
brain stem	at the center of posterior auricular sulcus.	The posterior auricular sulcus corresponds to brain stem.
soft palate	at the front lower side of brain stem.	
toothache point	at the inner side of brain stem, opposite soft palate.	
Helix		
external genital	near and at the same level as sympathetic.	
urethra	near and at the same level as bladder.	
lower section of rectum	near and at the same level as large intestine.	
anus	midway between lower section of rectum and urinary tract.	
ear apex	at the apex of the auricle.	
blind pile point	at the inner side of ear apex and below lowering pressure point.	
tonsil$_1$	outside ear apex and at a vertical line with tonsil in zone 8 of lobule.	
tonsil$_2$	midway between tonsil$_1$ and tonsil in the lobule area.	
tonsil$_3$	midway between tonsil$_2$ and tonsil in the lobule area.	
liver *yang*$_1$	at the upper rim of auricular tubercle.	
liver *yang*$_2$	at the lower rim of auricular tubercle.	

TABLE 4-1 (cont'd)

Ear Acupuncture Point	Anatomical Location	Remarks
Helix		
helix$_{1,2,3,4,5,6}$	at the lower edge of auricular tubercle is helix$_1$ and below tonsil is helix$_6$. Divide the distance between into four equal points and mark them top down as helix$_2$, helix$_3$, helix$_4$ and helix$_5$.	
minor occipital nerve	at 0.2 cm. inside of the upper rim of auricular tubercle.	
Posterior Auricle		
upper back	near the lower rim of the convex of posterior auricle.	
middle back	at the high point of the convex of posterior auricle.	
lower back	near the upper rim of the convex of posterior auricle.	
lowering pressure trough	at the upper ⅓ of the trough along the outer rim of the convex of posterior auricle.	
spinal cord$_1$	at the highest rim of ear root.	
spinal cord$_2$	at the lower rim of ear root.	
Others		
upper abdomen	at the lower inner rim of external acoustic meatus.	
lower abdomen	at the upper inner rim of external acoustic meatus.	
branch point	mid-point in a straight line between bladder and brain point.	

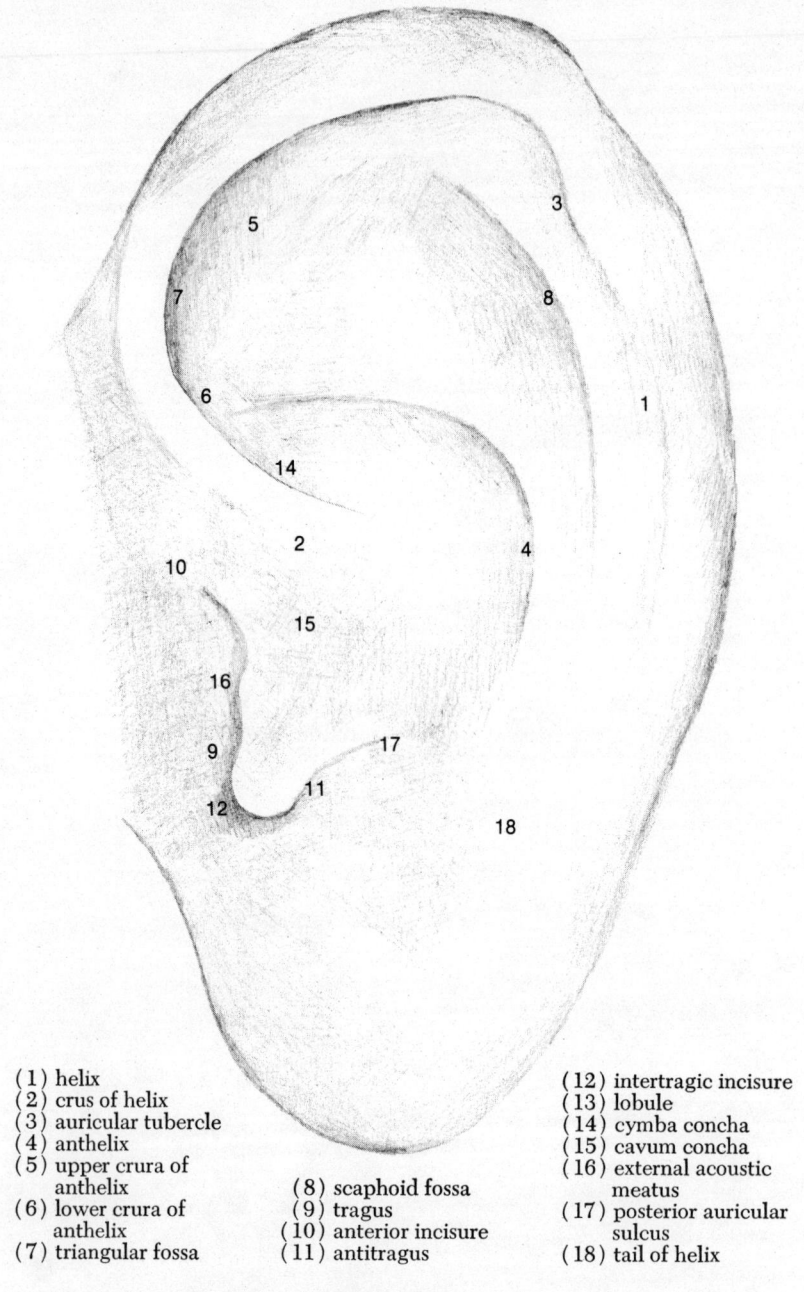

(1) helix
(2) crus of helix
(3) auricular tubercle
(4) anthelix
(5) upper crura of
     anthelix
(6) lower crura of
     anthelix
(7) triangular fossa

(8) scaphoid fossa
(9) tragus
(10) anterior incisure
(11) antitragus

(12) intertragic incisure
(13) lobule
(14) cymba concha
(15) cavum concha
(16) external acoustic
     meatus
(17) posterior auricular
     sulcus
(18) tail of helix

PLATE 1   Anatomical features of the auricle

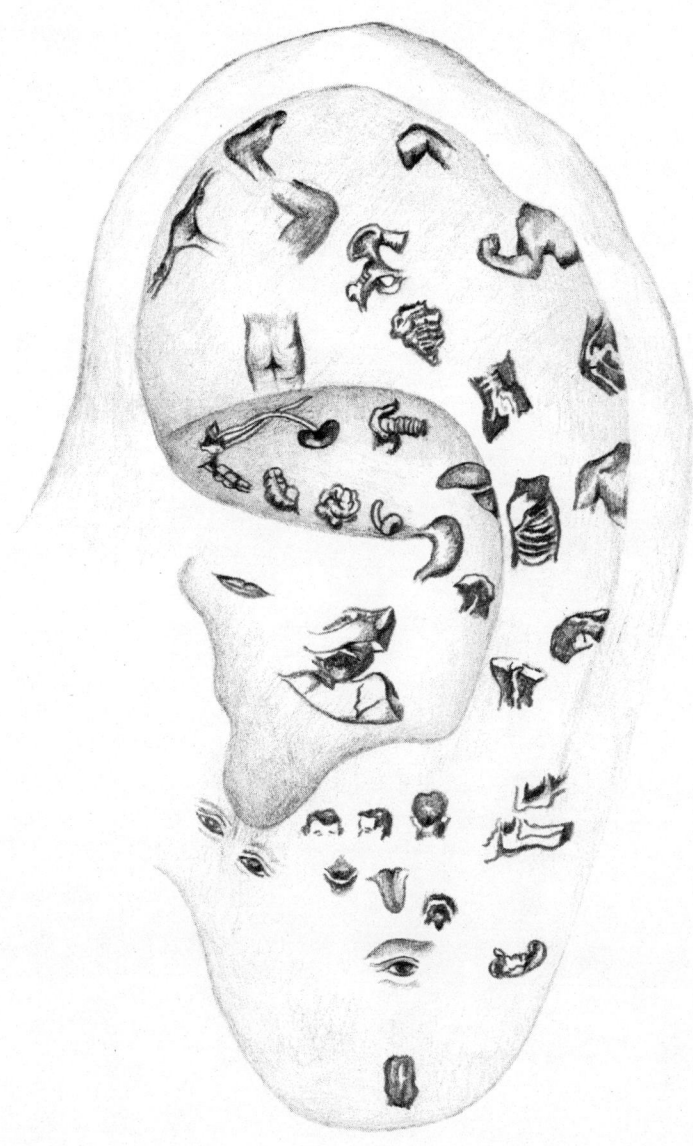

PLATE 2   Visual images of ear acupuncture points

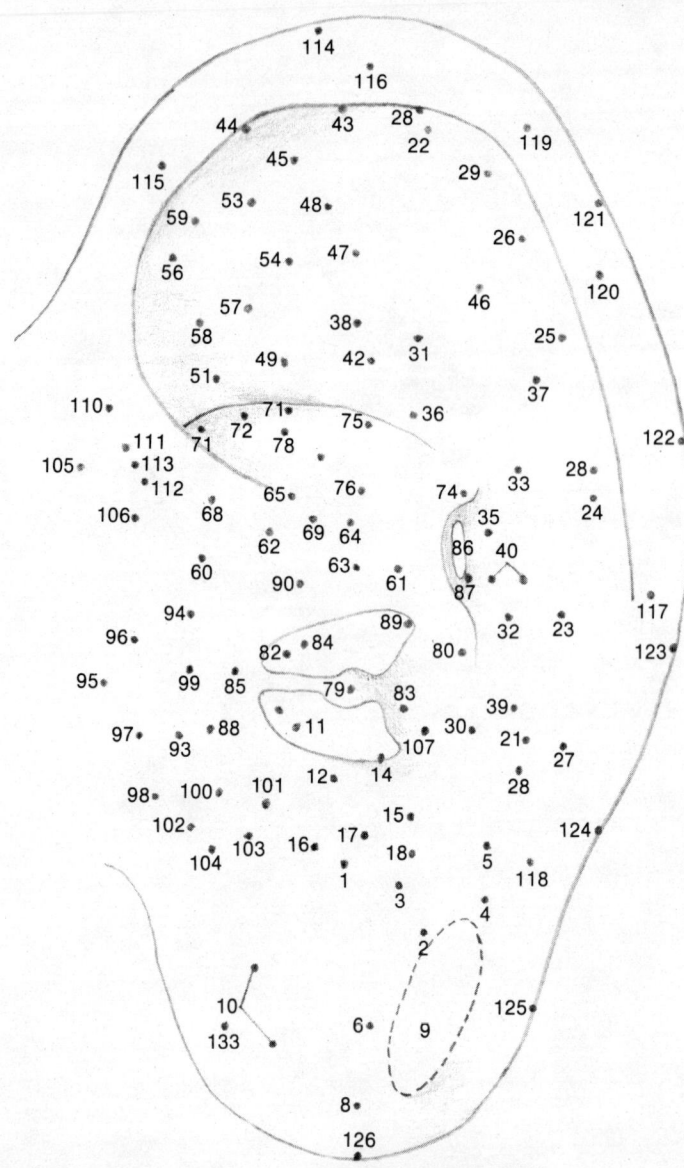

PLATE 3   Distribution of ear acupuncture points

PLATE 3   Distribution of ear acupuncture points

(1) lower palate
(2) upper palate
(3) tongue
(4) upper jowl
(5) lower jowl
(6) eye
(7) inner ear
(8) tonsil
(9) cheek area
(10) tooth extraction
      anaesthesia point
(11) parotid gland
(12) asthma
(13) testicle
(14) brain point
(15) occiput
(16) forehead
(17) greater *yang*
(18) apex
(19) lower dermis
(20) excitement point
(21) collarbone
(22) finger
(23) shoulder joint
(24) shoulder
(25) elbow
(26) wrist
(27) nephritis point
(28) appendix point
(29) urticaria point
(30) vertebra of neck
(31) sacral vertebra
(32) thoracic vertebra
(33) lumbar vertebra
(34) neck
(35) thorax
(36) abdomen
(37) outside abdomen
(38) heat point
(39) thyroid gland
(40) mammary gland
(41) appendix
      abdomen point
(42) lumbago point
(43) toe
(44) heel

(45) ankle joint
(46) knee
(47) hip joint
(48) knee joint
(49) buttock
(50) sympathetic
(51) sciatic nerve
(52) uterus
(53) *shen-men*
(54) pelvis cavum
(55) lowering pressure
      point
(56) asthma point
(57) thigh joint
(58) constipation point
(59) hepatitis point
(60) mouth
(61) stomach
(62) oesophagus
(63) cardia
(64) duodenum
(65) small intestine
(66) large intestine
(67) appendix
(68) diaphragm
(69) ear center
(70) bladder
(71) kidney
(72) ureter
(73) prostate
(74) liver
(75) pancreas gall
(76) pancreatitis point
(77) ascites point
(78) drunk point
(79) heart
(80) spleen
(81) lung
(82) bronchus
(83) tubercle point
(84) bronchiectasia
(85) trachea
(86) cirrhosis area
(87) hepatomegalia area
(88) triple warmer
(89) hepatitis area
(90) new eye point

(91) inner nose
(92) throat
(93) suprarenal point
(94) tragus apex
(95) outer nose
(96) thirst point
(97) hunger point
(98) high blood
      pressure point
(99) nose-ear purification
(100) internal secretion
(101) ovary
(102) eye_1
(103) eye_2
(104) rising pressure
       point
(105) outer ear
(106) cardiac point
(107) brain stem
(108) soft palate
(109) toothache point
(110) external genital
(111) urethra
(112) lower section
       of rectum
(113) anus
(114) ear apex
(115) blind pile point
(116) $tonsil_1$
(117) $tonsil_2$
(118) $tonsil_3$
(119) liver $yang_1$
(120) liver $yang_2$
(121) $helix_1$
(122) $helix_2$
(123) $helix_3$
(124) $helix_4$
(125) $helix_5$
(126) $helix_6$
(127) minor occipital
       nerve
(128) thyroid gland
(129) lower abdomen
(130) upper abdomen
(131) dumb gate
(132) nerve point
(133) neurasthenia point

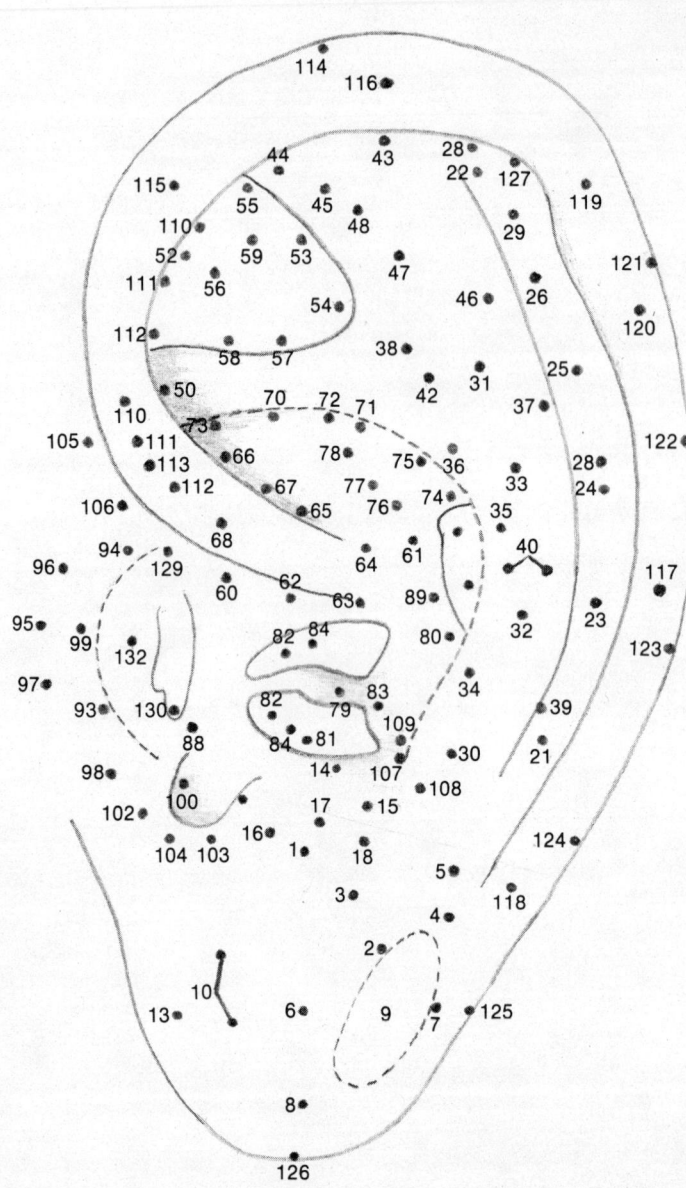

PLATE 4   Distribution of ear acupuncture points (plane)

PLATE 4   Distribution of ear acupuncture points (plane)

(1) lower palate
(2) upper palate
(3) tongue
(4) upper jowl
(5) lower jowl
(6) eye
(7) inner ear
(8) tonsil
(9) cheek area
(10) tooth extraction anaesthesia point
(11) parotid gland
(12) asthma
(13) testicle
(14) brain point
(15) occiput
(16) forehead
(17) greater *yang*
(18) apex
(19) lower dermis
(20) excitement point
(21) collarbone
(22) finger
(23) shoulder joint
(24) shoulder
(25) elbow
(26) wrist
(27) nephritis point
(28) appendix point
(29) urticaria point
(30) vertebra of neck
(31) sacral vertebra
(32) thoracic vertebra
(33) lumbar vertebra
(34) neck
(35) thorax
(36) abdomen
(37) outside abdomen
(38) heat point
(39) thyroid gland
(40) mammary gland
(41) appendix abdomen point
(42) lumbago point
(43) toe
(44) heel

(45) ankle joint
(46) knee
(47) hip joint
(48) knee joint
(49) buttock
(50) sympathetic
(51) sciatic nerve
(52) uterus
(53) *shen-men*
(54) pelvis cavum
(55) lowering pressure point
(56) asthma point
(57) thigh joint
(58) constipation point
(59) hepatitis point
(60) mouth
(61) stomach
(62) oesophagus
(63) cardia
(64) duodenum
(65) small intestine
(66) large intestine
(67) appendix
(68) diaphragm
(69) ear center
(70) bladder
(71) kidney
(72) ureter
(73) prostate
(74) liver
(75) pancreas gall
(76) pancreatitis point
(77) ascites point
(78) drunk point
(79) heart
(80) spleen
(81) lung
(82) bronchus
(83) tubercle point
(84) bronchiectasia
(85) trachea
(86) cirrhosis area
(87) hepatomegalia area
(88) triple warmer
(89) hepatitis area
(90) new eye point

(91) inner nose
(92) throat
(93) suprarenal point
(94) tragus apex
(95) outer nose
(96) thirst point
(97) hunger point
(98) high blood pressure point
(99) nose-ear purification
(100) internal secretion
(101) ovary
(102) eye_1
(103) eye_2
(104) rising pressure point
(105) outer ear
(106) cardiac point
(107) brain stem
(108) soft palate
(109) toothache point
(110) external genital
(111) urethra
(112) lower section of rectum
(113) anus
(114) ear apex
(115) blind pile point
(116) $tonsil_1$
(117) $tonsil_2$
(118) $tonsil_3$
(119) liver $yang_1$
(120) liver $yang_2$
(121) $helix_1$
(122) $helix_2$
(123) $helix_3$
(124) $helix_4$
(125) $helix_5$
(126) $helix_6$
(127) minor occipital nerve
(128) thyroid gland
(129) lower abdomen
(130) upper abdomen
(131) dumb gate
(132) nerve point
(133) neurasthenia point

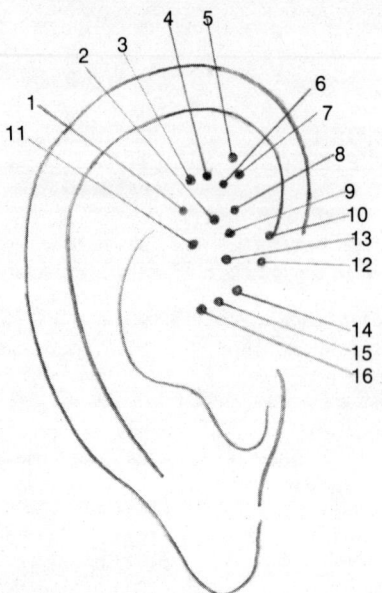

(1) pelvis cavum
(2) thigh joint
(3) *shen-men*
(4) hepatitis point
(5) lowering pressure
      point
(6) asthma point
(7) uterus
(8) constipation point
(9) sciatic nerve
(10) sympathetic
(11) buttock
(12) prostate
(13) bladder
(14) large intestine
(15) appendix
(16) small intestine

PLATE 5   Distribution of ear acupuncture points in triangular fossa

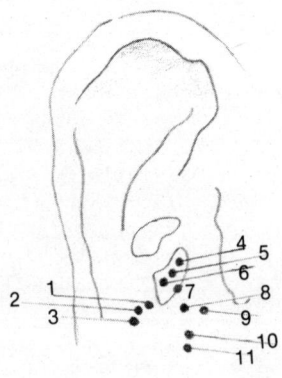

(1) soft palate
(2) brain stem
(3) toothache point
(4) bronchi
(5) tubercle point
(6) bronchiectasia
(7) lung point
(8) excitement point
(9) dermis
(10) testicle
(11) parotid gland

PLATE 6   Distribution of ear acupuncture points in antitragus

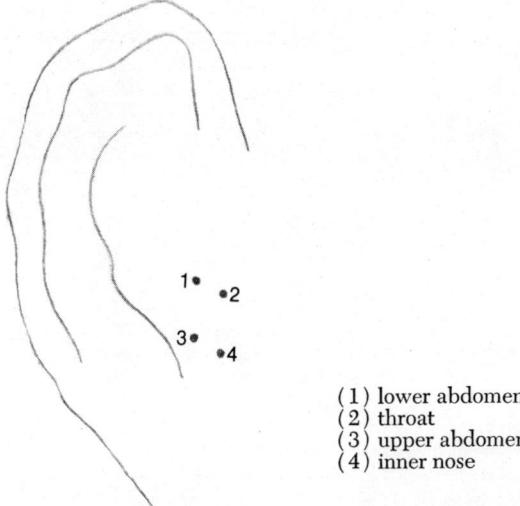

(1) lower abdomen
(2) throat
(3) upper abdomen
(4) inner nose

PLATE 7   Distribution of ear acupuncture points in tragus

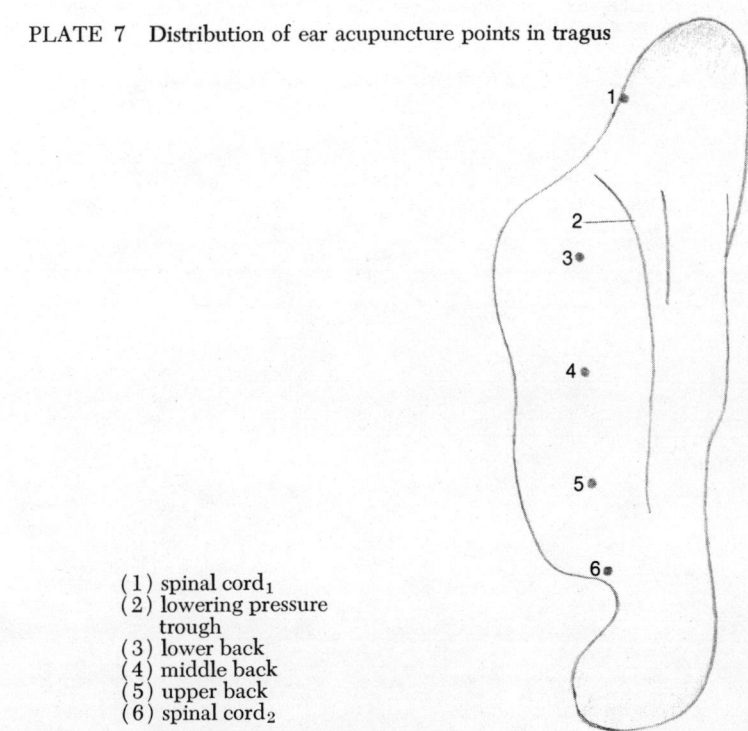

(1) spinal cord$_1$
(2) lowering pressure
   trough
(3) lower back
(4) middle back
(5) upper back
(6) spinal cord$_2$

PLATE 8   Distribution of ear acupuncture points at posterior auricle

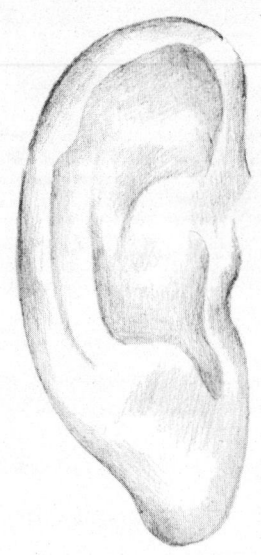 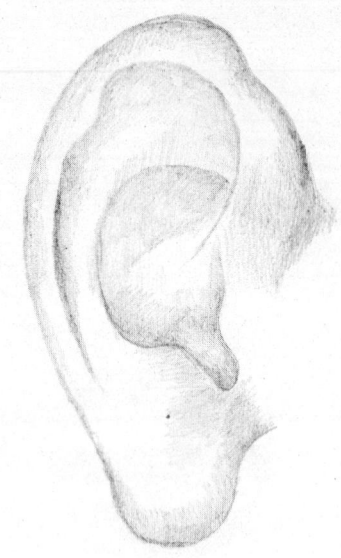

(1) stomach ulcer—white point with red rim in stomach area

(2) hepatomegalia—white flake-shaped swelling in liver area

PLATE 9-1   Diagnosis of the auricle

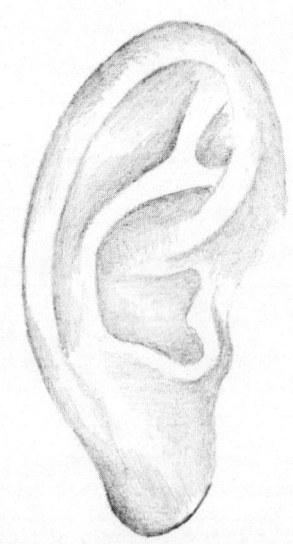 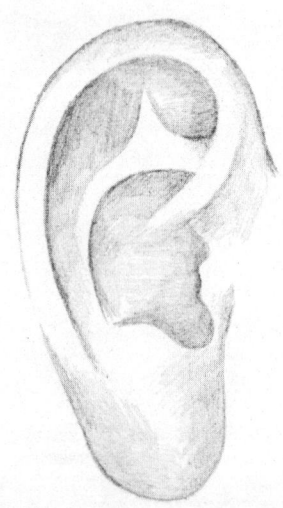

(1) skin disease—skin peeling in lung area

(2) gynecological disease—hives or skin peeling in uterus area

PLATE 9-2   Diagnosis of the auricle

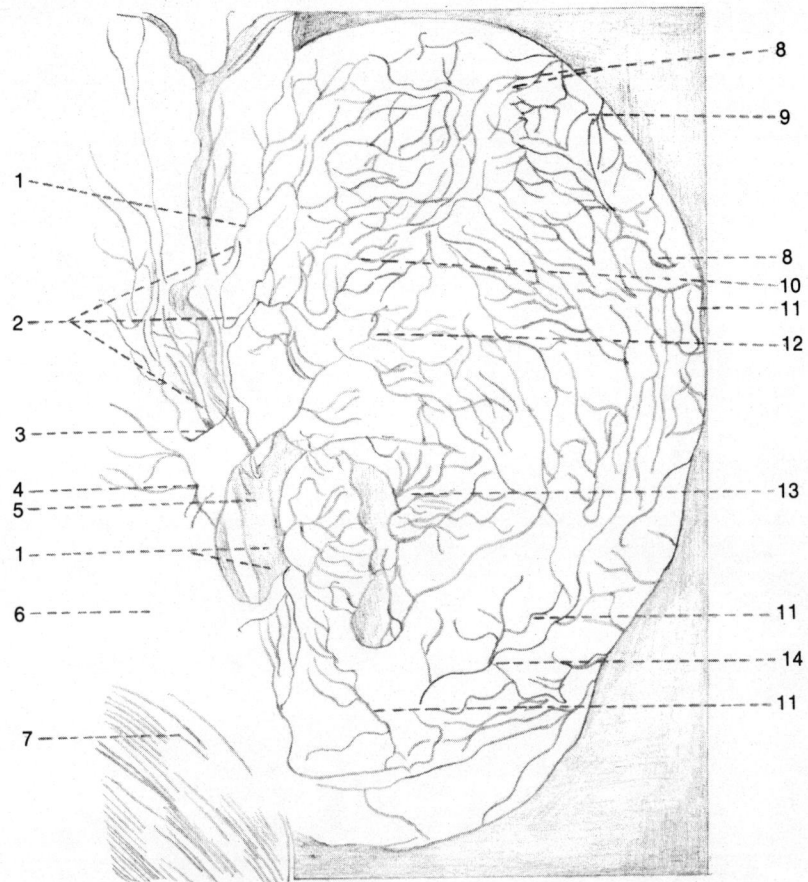

(1) auricular anterior branch of superficial temporal artery

(2) auricular anterior branch of auriculotemporal nerve

(3) auriculotemporal nerve

(4) auricular anterior ligament

(5) superficial temporal artery and vein

(6) parotid gland

(7) platysma myoides

(8) connective branch of auricular posterior artery and minor occipital nerve

(9) auricular anterior branch of minor occipital nerve

(10) connective branch of auricular posterior artery

(11) auricular anterior branch of major auricular nerve

(12) anterior connective sub-branch of auricular posterior branch of facial nerve

(13) anterior connective sub-branch of auricular branch of vagus nerve

(14) auricular anterior branch of auricular posterior artery

PLATE 10   Anatomy of anterior auricle

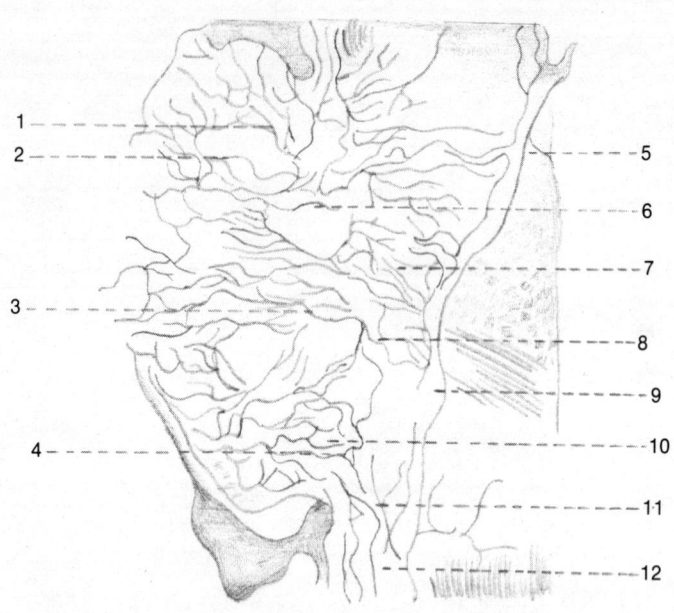

(1) auricular posterior
    branch of minor
    occipital nerve
(2) auricular branch of
    auricular posterior
    artery
(3) auricular posterior
    branch of major
    auricular nerve
(4) auricular anterior
    branch of major
    auricular nerve
(5) minor occipital
    nerve
(6) auricular posterior
    branch of facial
    nerve

(7) auricular posterior
    muscle
(8) auricular posterior
    branch of facial
    nerve
(9) auricular posterior
    vein
(10) auricular anterior
    branch of auricular
    posterior artery
(11) major auricular
    nerve
(12) auricular posterior
    artery

PLATE 11   Anatomy of posterior auricle (superficial level)

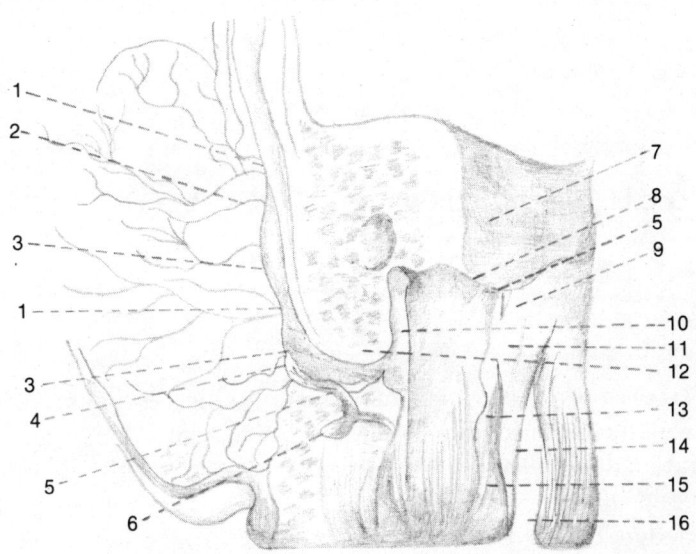

(1) auricular anterior
    branch of facial
    nerve
(2) auricular posterior
    branch of facial
    nerve
(3) auricular anterior
    branch of vagus
    nerve
(4) auricular branch of
    facial nerve
(5) auricular branch of
    vagus nerve
(6) auricular posterior
    artery

(7) petrosa
(8) cervical vein nest
(9) vagus nerve
(10) facial nerve
(11) hypoglossus nerve
(12) mastoid
(13) accessory nerve
(14) nodosum ganglion
(15) internal carotid
    artery
(16) superior cervical
    ganglion

PLATE 12   Anatomy of posterior auricle (deeper level)

CHAPTER 5

The Function of Ear Acupuncture Points Commonly Used in Treatment

"To discover truth we always start with perceptual knowledge of the material world, develop it into rational knowledge, and then test rational knowledge in the material world. In other words, we must repeat the pattern from practice to knowledge and from knowledge back to practice innumerable times before truth is obtained."[1] The same is also true with the exploration of the function of ear acupuncture points. In numerous clinical practices we came to realize that the function of acupuncture points must be studied first from its particularity and then from its universality.

In our exploration of the two aspects of the function of ear acupuncture points, we felt that their therapeutic importance and effect should not be overlooked. Correct recognition and handling of contradictions (unity of opposites) between their particularity and universality would have great effect in curing diseases. We are convinced that most ear acupuncture points not only have the normal function of their anatomical features in modern medical science but also have the rich significance contained in the theory of vessels and meridians and the viscera theory of traditional Chinese medicine.

---

[1] This and most other quotations in this book are taken from Mao Tse-tung's two philosophical essays "On Practice" and "On Contradiction."

We have followed Chairman Mao's teaching, "practice, knowledge, more practice, more knowledge." On the basis of Chinese and Western medical theories, we carried out numerous experiments in exploring the physiological function of ear acupuncture points and their mutual relations. The following is our preliminary analysis of the function of ear acupuncture points:

Heart: The heart has the function of making mind tranquil and spirit peaceful, regulating blood circulation, and calming anxiety. This acupuncture point can thus be used to cure cardiac diseases, palpitation of heart, shortness in breath, and chest pains. The heart controls blood vessels, so it can be used to treat diseases of the cardiovascular system. It controls clearness in the head and its function is related to perspiration, so that it can be used to cure nightsweat, insomnia, excessive dreams, amnesia, neurasthenia, and mental diseases. The orifice of heart is tongue, and its vessels and meridians pass by both sides of the throat, so that this point can be used to cure chronic pharyngitis, hoarse voice, painful and inflamed tongue, and stomatitis.

Liver: The liver has the function of benefiting gall, dispelling evil spirits, regulating blood circulation, improving eyesight, and strengthening the stomach. This acupuncture point is used primarily for curing acute and chronic hepatitis, inflammation of gall bladder, jaundice, and dermatophiliasis. "Evil winds and dizzy spells originate in the liver." The liver controls muscles; thus it can be used to cure fainting, convulsion, paralysis caused by accidental damage to blood vessels in brain, muscular asthenia, and sprains. Liver stores blood; thus it can be used to cure blood diseases, hemorrhagic diseases, and iron deficiency anemia. The orifice of liver is the eye, so the liver acupuncture point can be used to cure eye diseases. Blood vessels from the liver link the stomach, so it can be used in treating diseases of the digestive system. Liver controls dispersion and its pulse air concentrates in the armpit, so that it can be used for relieving chest heaviness, generalized sourness and pain, abdominal distention, and depression.

Spleen: The spleen manages circulation and digestion, modifies blood, nourishes muscle, and strengthens air. This acupuncture point is used primarily to cure indigestion, gastritis, and gastroduodenic ulcers. The spleen controls blood, so that it can be used for treating bleeding ailments, blood diseases, and anemia. It manages muscle and the efficacy of its function is reflected in lips, so that it can be used in curing muscle dystrophy, muscular asthenia, muscular atrophy caused by a variety of factors, stomatitis, and ulcer. It is also effective in treating rectal prolapse caused by the lowering of middle air, prolapse of internal organs, and chronic diarrhea caused by splenatrophy.

Lung: Lungs manage air, control breathing, oxygenate blood and promote its circulation, assist urination, compensate insufficiency, and regulate body temperature. This acupuncture point cures diseases of the respiratory system, such as tuberculosis, cough, asthma, and edema caused by obstruction of the large and small circulatory system. Lungs control the surface area of human body including skin and hair, so that it is effective in curing influenza, nightsweat, involuntary perspiration, and a number of skin diseases. The lung artery extends to the throat, so it can cure hoarseness and laryngitis. Lungs and the large intestine are connected by the artery, so that this acupunture point can be used for treating enteritis and diarrhea. It is also effective in treating stomatitis and lip ulcer. In ear acupuncture anaesthesia, it is the main point to kill pain during incision.

Kidney: Kidneys function to strengthen *yang* air, nourish sperm, toughen lumbar vertebrae, aid brain tissue, assist urination, and sharpen eyes and ears. This acupuncture point is primarily used in treating nephritis, kidney pyelitis, inefficiency of kidneys, cystitis, and diseases of the reproductory system (such as impotency, spermatorrhea, gynaecological diseases). The orifice of kidneys is the ear, and since kidneys control bones and the essence of bones is the pupil, this acupuncture point can be used to treat deafness, tinnitus aurium, lessening hearing power, eye diseases, and pain caused by broken bones. "Teeth are the residue of bones," kidneys store essence (*ching*), and essence produces marrow. Brain is the sea of marrow, so this acupuncture point can be used for treating loose teeth, tooth bleeding, mental diseases, diseases of the nerve system, neurasthenia, and headache. The flower of kidneys is hair, so it is also effective in curing losing hair and alopecia areata. In Chinese medicine, "kidneys are the innate essence." Kidneys and bladder, intimately related, are the root of all physical activities. This acupuncture point can be used to assist digestion of food, and to cure lack of appetite and reinvigorate all kinds of chronic and impotent syndromes. At the same time, because the orifice of kidneys is *erh yin* it can cure constipation.

Large Intestine: The large intestine discharges dregs, so this acupuncture point is used to cure dysenteria, entritis, diarrhea, appendicitis, constipation, and loose bowels. Large and small intestines are subordinate to the stomach, and all belong to the digestive system, so that it is also effective in treating indigestion. The large intestine and lungs are intimately connected by meridians, so that it can be used for curing diseases of the respiratory system.

Small Intestine: The small intestine manages digestion and separates nutriment from excrement. Its vessels link the stomach. This acupuncture point is used for curing diarrhea, indigestion, diminishing absorbing function of stomach and intestines, abdominal distention, and intestinal tubercles. The vessel of small intestine links the heart, so this acupuncture point can be used for treating cardiac diseases such as palpitation and shortness of breath. The vessel of small intestine controls ailments of succus and extends upward to surround the neck, so this point is used for treating milk insufficiency (galactozemia), sore throat, and swollen neck.

Stomach: The stomach manages receiving and digesting food and is intimately related to the spleen. This acupuncture point is used for curing stomach ulcer, chronic gastritis, gastric nerve pain, indigestion, loss of appetite, and excessive or insufficient gastric acid. The stomach enjoys downward circulation, so to balance the stomach cures nausea and vomiting caused by upward regression of stomach air. The vessel from the stomach extends to the teeth, passes the hair, and reaches the forehead, so it can be used for treating fore headache, diseases of the nervous system (such as epilepsy, hysteria, schizophrenia, and insomnia), and toothache.

Gall Bladder: The gall bladder stores gall and is intimately related to liver. This acupuncture point can be used for curing gall bladder inflammation, ascarid in the gall bladder, gallstones, and hepatogenic icterus. The vessel from the gall bladder extends via neck to the temple, reaches the posterior auricle, enters the middle ear, and exits at the anterior auricle. Thus, this acupuncture point can be used for treating deafness, tinnitus aurium, excessive dreams, migraine headache, and stiff neck.

Bladder: The bladder stores liquid (urine) and is intimately related to kidneys. This acupuncture point can be used for treating acute and chronic cystitis, kidney pyelitis, glomerutitis, prostatitis, bed-wetting, frequent urge to urinate, uriesthesis, lack of control of bladder, and uroschesis. The vessel from the bladder extends via the rear of the thigh, hip, rear lumbar, to the rear of the neck, and enters brain tissue, so that this point is also used to cure migraine headache, lumbar vertebral pain, sciatic neuralgia, neurasthenia, and insomnia.

Triple Warmer: The triple warmer synthesizes all the functions of five viscera and six bowels, so that this acupuncture point can be used for treating diseases of the circulatory system, the reproductory system, heart, and thorax, axilla pain, shortness of breath, indigestion, anemia, hepatitis, abdominal distention, obstruction in absorption, and peritonitis. The triple warmer promotes liquid circulation, so it cures hydrops caused by a number of factors. The vessel from the triple warmer spreads in the outer section of the arm, so that it can be used for treating arm pain.

Shen-men: This acupuncture point can be used for tranquilizing the mind, killing pains, and often treating insomnia, restlessness, common mental disorder, excessive sensitivity, and sundry pains. It is an important acupuncture point for anaesthesia. It can reduce fever, neutralize poison, and cure inflammatory diseases. It can also lower temper, relieve cough, cure dry cough (not to be applied to the type with excessive sputum), and bronchial asthma. It is effective in harmonizing liver, quelling wind, curing epilepsy, and high blood pressure.

Sympathetic: This acupuncture point is used in curing diseases caused by neuro-vegetative disequilibrium. It has a stronger effect in killing pain and relieving contraction in intestinal organs, such as griping pains caused by ulcers, ascarid in the gall bladder, gallstones, and urinary lithiasis. It may cause dilatation of blood vessels and is thus often used in treating pulselessness, vasculitis and cardiogmus caused by narrowing and spasm of arteries and veins. It can also be used in curing irregular heart rhythm, tachycardia, premature contraction, nightsweat, and involuntary perspiration. It is also effective in treating eye diseases. Finally, it is a major acupuncture anaesthesia point in operations on chest and abdomen.

Suprarenal Gland: This acupuncture point represents the suprarenal gland and the suprarenal cortex and has the function of regulating the suprarenal gland and hormones produced by the suprarenal cortex. It is used for treating inflammations and relieving hypersensitivity, rheumatism, infection, and shock. It has the effect of dilating or contracting blood vessels and therefore can be used in curing high or low blood pressure, pulselessness, vascular inflammation, and capillary hemorrhage. It can reduce fever or heat caused by unknown factors. This acupuncture point can also be used for halting cough, relieving asthma, and curing skin diseases.

Internal Secretion: This acupuncture point represents the internal secretion system. It is often used in treating diseases caused by disorderly internal secretion, relieving hypersensitivity, and rheumatism. It can also be used in curing certain skin diseases, diseases of the urinary and reproductory systems, gynemetrical diseases, diseases of blood vessels, obstruction in the absorptive system of the stomach and intestines, and malaria.

Dermis: This acupuncture point represents the outer cortex of the cerebrum and can be used in regulating excitement and restraint of cerebral cortex. All kinds of syndromes caused by excitement or loss of restraint of cerebral cortex can be treated. It can also be used in curing visceral prolapse. Finally, it can restore tranquility, kill pains, counteract inflammation, reduce swelling, halt sweating, and treat shock.

Occiput: It is commonly used in treating diseases of the nervous system and cerebral irritation, such as spasm, opisthotonos, trismus, stiff neck, prolapse of occiput, and shock. It is rather effective in preventing and treating car sickness and sea sickness. It can also be used in treating presbyopia and skin diseases. Finally, it has a certain effect in counteracting inflammation, restoring tranquility, killing pains, halting cough, and stopping asthma.

Brain Stem: This acupuncture point represents the medulla oblongata and the brain stem. Its function is for regulating disorder and harmonizing wind. It is effective in treating cerebral irritation, such as opisthotonos and spasm. It can be used for strengthening the brain and invigorating the spirit and therefore for curing the underdeveloped cerebrum, sequela of brain trauma, and sequela of meningitis. Finally, it can be used for emergency treatment of shock, treatment of hypersensitivity, pain killing, and haemostasia.

Brain Point: This acupuncture point represents the pituitary gland and can be used for treating diseases caused by malfunction of the pituitary gland, such as dwarfism, hypertrophic limbs, diabetes insipidus, excessive menstruation, and metrorrhagia. It is also effective in stopping asthma and inducing tranquility and sleep. Furthermore, it has a certain effect in treating bed-wetting and vascular inflammation.

Pancreatitis Point: It is commonly used in treating pancreatitis, indigestion and diabetes mellitus. It is also effective in curing migraine headache.

Uterus: This acupuncture point is used in treating inflammation of pelvis cavum, inflammation of uteral lining, metrorrhagia, irregular menstruation, leukorrhea, postpartum uteralgia, obstruction in sexual function, testitis, and secondary testitis. It can also be used to induce early delivery.

Forehead: This acupuncture point has the effect of inducing tranquility and killing pains. It is used in treating frontal headache, neurasthenia, insomnia, excessive dreams, nasitis, and nasosinuitis.

Temple: It is used in treating migraine headache, sleeping sickness, and night urination caused by sleeping sickness.

Parotid Gland: It is used in treating parotitis, obstruction in parotid gland, and skin diseases.

Asthma: It is effective in regulating the central system of respiration, controlling hypersensitivity, and stopping itching. It is commonly used for treating cough, asthma, difficult breathing, short breath, suffocating chest, and allergic itching.

Testicle: It is used in treating obstruction in sexual function, testitis, and secondary testitis.

Ovary: It is used for treating obstruction in sexual function, irregular menstruation, ovaritis, inflammation in the Fallopian tube (oviduct), and infertility.

Excitement Point: It is used for treating sleeping sickness and bed-wetting caused by sleeping sickness.

Ascites Point: It is used for treating cirrhosis and abdominal dropsy, and flatulence caused by assorted ailments of kidneys.

Throat: It is used for treating acute and chronic pharyngitis and laryngitis, hoarseness, uvular edema, tonsilitis, loss of voice, bronchitis, and bronchial asthma.

Inner Nose: It is used for treating a variety of rhinitis, nasosinuitis, nasovestibular ulcer, furuncle in nasal passage, and influenza.

Outer Nose: It is used for treating nasal furuncle and rosacea.

Tragus Apex: It is used for blood-letting to reduce fever, reduce inflammation and treat common inflammation. It is also effective in inducing tranquility and killing pains.

Diaphragm: It is used for treating diaphragmatic muscle spasm, blood diseases, and skin diseases. It is somewhat effective in curing visceral bleeding and hemoptysis.

Ear Center: The function of this point is basically the same as the triple warmer.

Ear Apex: Primarily for blood-letting. Bloodletting two or three drops each time can reduce fever, lower blood pressure, counteract inflammation, reduce ammonemia, and cure delirium caused by liver ailment. It is also very effective in inducing tranquility and killing pains.

Lower Section of Rectum: It is used for treating internal and external hemorrhoids, rectal prolapse, incontinence of excrement, and rectal discomfort caused by diarrhea.

Urethra: It is used for treating urethritis, lack of control of bladder, and urethrostenosis.

External Genital: It is used for treating phallitis, rashes in scrotum, impotency, and pains in loins and thighs.

Tonsil$_{1-4}$*:* It is used for treating tonsillitis, pharyngitis and laryngitis.

Helix$_{1-6}$*:* It is used for counteracting inflammation, reducing fever, relieving swelling, and lowering blood pressure. By letting blood from these acupuncture points, tonsillitis and high blood pressure can be cured.

Liver Yang$_{1,2}$*:* It is used for treating chronic hepatitis. It is also effective in curing spreading infectious hepatitis and prolonged high level of transaminase.

Eye$_1$*:* It is used for treating acute and chronic glaucoma and optic atrophy.

Eye$_2$*:* It is used for treating a variety of eye diseases.

Eye: It is commonly used for treating a variety of eye diseases such as acute conjunctivitis, stye, chalazion, keratitis, pterygium, and zig-zags in front of the eyes.

New Eye: It is used for treating zig-zags in front of the eyes and ailment behind the eyes.

Outer Ear: For treating deafness, tinnitus aurium, lessening hearing power, auricular frostbite and infection.

Inner Ear: For treating deafness, tinnitus aurium, lessening hearing power, otitis media, furuncle at outer ear, and auditory dizziness.

Tooth Extraction Anaesthesia Point: For anaesthesia in tooth extraction and pains caused by decayed teeth.

Upper and Lower Palate: For treating mouth ulcers, peridontal inflammation and for anaesthesia in mending a broken palate.

Upper and Lower Jowl: For killing toothache, anaesthesia in tooth extraction, treating lower jowl rheumatism, and jowl lymphadenitis.

Cheek Area: For treating trigeminal neuralgia, parotitis, facial nervous spasm, facial nervous paralysis, acne and furuncle in cheek area.

Collarbone: For killing pains in fixing collarbone fracture, shoulder periarthritis, and narrowness of carotid artery.

Shoulder Joint: For treating strained shoulder joint and shoulder periarthritis.

Shoulder: Its function is the same as shoulder joint.

Elbow: For treating strained elbow joint and sore upper arm.

Wrist: For treating strained wrist joint and pain in the gastric nerve.

Finger: For treating strained finger joint, dactylitis, and frost-bite.

Neck Vertebra: For treating generation or degeneration of neck vertebra and strained neck.

Thoracic Vertebra: For treating generation or degeneration of thoracic vertebra.

Lumbar and Sacral Vertebra: For treating generation or degeneration of lumbar and sacral vertebra and strained lumbar and sacral vertebra.

Neck: For treating strained neck, hyper- or hypo-thyroidism, and carotid arteriostenosis.

Thorax: For treating thorax diseases, intercostal neuralgia, chest pain, and chest heaviness.

Abdomen: For treating abdominal diseases, diseases of the digestive system, and gynemetrical diseases.

Outside Abdomen: This acupuncture point is more commonly used for diagnosis. If there is the *yang* reaction in the gall bladder point or the kidney point and this point also shows pain reaction, then the possibility for gallstone or kidneystone is much greater.

Heat Point: It is effective for killing pains and dilating blood vessels and particularly effective for treating acute strained lumbar, pulselessness, and vascular inflammation.

Mammary Gland: For treating mastitis, no milk, insufficient milk, and proliferation of mammary gland ducts.

Knee Joint: For treating knee rheumatism, strained knee joint and killing pains caused by broken kneecap bone.

Toe: For treating strained toe joint, frostbite, and inflammation.

Sciatic Nerve: For treating sciatic neuralgia, sciatic neuritis, paralysis of lower limbs, and polio.

Upper, Middle, Lower Back: For treating backache, skin diseases, and stopping itching.

Lowering Pressure Trough: Primarily for blood-letting in order to lower blood pressure.

Spinal Cord: For treating amyotrophic lateral sclerosis and a variety of paralysis.

Minor Occipital Nerve: This acupuncture point has a pain-killing effect. It is used for treating cerebral blood vessel spasm, sequela of brain trauma, headache, dizziness, partial paralysis caused by hemorrhage, and head numbness caused by nervous functional disorder.

CHAPTER 6

Tables Listing
Ear Acupuncture Points
for Treating Common Diseases

TABLE 6-1
Digestive System

Diseases	Primary Acupuncture Points	Secondary Acupuncture Points
*nausea; vomiting	stomach, *shen-men*, occiput, sympathetic	dermis, oesophagus
acute & chronic gastritis	stomach, sympathetic, *shen-men*, spleen	abdomen, lung
*functional disease of gastric nerves	stomach, liver, sympathetic, *shen-men*	duodenum, minor occipital nerve
stomach ulcer	stomach, sympathetic, *shen-men*, spleen, lung	dermis, duodenum
duodenal ulcer	duodenum, sympathetic, *shen-men*	stomach, lung
*gastric spasm	stomach, sympathetic, ear center	upper abdomen, *shen-men*
prolapse of stomach	stomach, sympathetic, dermis	liver
chronic gall bladder inflammation	gall, liver, sympathetic, lung	internal secretion
chronic pancreatitis	pancreas, internal secretion, sympathetic, *shen-men*, pancreatitis point	

Note: Asterisk (*) indicates high effectiveness, with curing rate above 90%.

53

TABLE 6-1 (cont'd)

Diseases	Primary Acupuncture Points	Secondary Acupuncture Points
°diaphragmatic spasm	diaphragm, shen-men, dermis, ear center	
°diarrhea	large intestine, small intestine, sympathetic, spleen	
abdominal distention	small intestine, large intestine, stomach, sympathetic	abdomen, triple warmer
°enteritis	large intestine, sympathetic, small intestine, lung	
°indigestion	small intestine, stomach, pancreas-gall, spleen	
°intestinal colic	small intestine, sympathetic, ear center, lower abdomen	
gastric & intestinal disorder	stomach, large intestine, small intestine, sympathetic, spleen	triple warmer
allergic colitis	large intestine, internal secretion, sympathetic, lung, small intestine	
°constipation	large intestine, lower section of rectum, dermis, constipation	sympathetic, spleen
alcoholism	occiput, forehead, drunk point, minor occipital nerve	

TABLE 6-2

Respiratory System

Diseases	Primary Acupuncture Points	Secondary Acupuncture Points
cough	asthma, suprarenal gland, throat, occiput, lung	shen-men
chest heaviness	sympathetic, heart, thorax, lung, asthma	
°chest pain	corresponding area, shen-men	
common cold; influenza	inner nose, suprarenal gland, forehead, lung	
bronchitis	bronchus, shen-men, asthma, suprarenal gland	sympathetic, occiput

Note: Asterisk (°) indicates high effectiveness, with curing rate above 90%.

TABLE 6-2 (cont'd)

Diseases	Primary Acupuncture Points	Secondary Acupuncture Points
asthma	sympathetic, *shen-men,* asthma, suprarenal gland	lung, occiput
whooping cough	bronchus, suprarenal gland, asthma, sympathetic	occiput
pneumonia	lung, thorax, suprarenal gland, internal secretion	dermis
broncho-pneumonia	bronchus, sympathetic, asthma, suprarenal gland	occiput, internal secretion

TABLE 6-3

Circulatory System

Diseases	Primary Acupuncture Points	Secondary Acupuncture Points
high blood pressure	lowering pressure point, sympathetic, *shen-men,* heart, ear apex blood-letting	
low blood pressure	sympathetic, heart, suprarenal gland, dermis	
*pulselessness	sympathetic, heat point, kidney, heart, suprarenal gland, liver, corresponding area, dermis	
tachycardia	heart, sympathetic, *shen-men,* small intestine, dermis	
myocarditis	heart, sympathetic, *shen-men,* small intestine, spleen	
iron-deficiency anemia	liver, spleen, internal secretion, diaphragm, stomach, small intestine	
granulocyto-penia	liver, spleen, heart, kidney, internal secretion, suprarenal gland	occiput, diaphragm, sympathetic
premature contraction	heart, sympathetic, small intestine, dermis, cardiac point	
coronary thrombosis	heart, sympathetic, internal secretion, suprarenal gland	small intestine, kidney dermis

Note: Asterisk (*) indicates high effectiveness, with curing rate above 90%.

TABLE 6-4

Nervous System

Diseases	Primary Acupuncture Points	Secondary Acupuncture Points
*headache; dizziness	occiput, forehead, *shen-men*, dermis, minor occipital nerve	
*insomnia	*shen-men*, kidney, occiput, heart	
excessive dreams	*shen-men*, kidney, occiput, heart, stomach	triple warmer
*migraine	temple, minor occipital nerve, *shen-men*, kidney, dermis	
trigeminal neuralgia	cheek, upper & lower jowl, *shen-men*, occiput	outer ear, minor occipital nerve
facial nerve paralysis	cheek area, minor occipital nerve, eye, mouth, dermis	liver, occiput
*intercostal neuralgia	thorax, occiput, *shen-men*	
sciatica	sciatic, *shen-men*, kidney	
sciatic neuritis	sciatic, kidney, *shen-men*, occiput, suprarenal gland	
*sequela of brain trauma	kidney, brain stem, occiput, *shen-men*, forehead, dermis	heart, minor occipital nerve
sequela of meningitis	kidney, brain stem, occiput, *shen-men*, dermis	stomach, heart, minor occipital nerve
epilepsy	*shen-men*, occiput, heart, stomach, dermis	minor occipital nerve
*neurasthenia	kidney, *shen-men*, occiput, heart, stomach	dermis
hysteria	*shen-men*, occiput, heart, stomach, brain stem	dermis
schizophrenia	kidney, *shen-men*, occiput, heart, stomach	brain stem, dermis, minor occipital nerve
hysteric paralysis	dermis, *shen-men*, occiput, heart, corresponding area	stomach, kidney, minor occipital nerve
hysteric aphasia	brain point, occiput, heart, *shen-men*, kidney	dermis
facial nerve spasm	cheek area, *shen-men*, dermis, temple, liver	minor occipital nerve
shock	suprarenal gland, occiput, heart, brain point, dermis	

Note: Asterisk (*) indicates high effectiveness, with curing rate above 90%.

TABLE 6-4 (cont'd)

Diseases	Primary Acupuncture Points	Secondary Acupuncture Points
nervous excessive drinking	internal secretion, dermis, *shen-men,* kidney, thirst point, brain point	
sequela of polio	corresponding area, *shen-men,* suprarenal gland, internal secretion	dermis, occiput
excessive sweating	sympathetic, lung, internal secretion, occiput, suprarenal gland	
*heat stroke	occiput, heart, dermis, suprarenal gland	minor occipital nerve

TABLE 6-5

Urinary and Reproductory System

Diseases	Primary Acupuncture Points	Secondary Acupuncture Points
frequent urge to urinate	bladder, kidney, *shen-men,* urethra, dermis	
uriesthesis	bladder, kidney, *shen-men,* urethra	
uroschesis	kidney, bladder, sympathetic, external genital, dermis	
bed-wetting	bladder, branch point, excitement point, occiput, kidney	brain point
*cystitis	bladder, kidney, sympathetic, occiput, suprarenal gland	
kidney pyelitis	kidney, bladder, sympathetic, liver, internal secretion, suprarenal gland	spleen
urinary lithiasis	ureter, kidney, sympathetic, dermis, bladder	
acute nephritis	kidney, bladder, sympathetic, liver, internal secretion, suprarenal gland	spleen
impotency	uterus, external genital, testicle, internal secretion, kidney	
testitis	testicle, internal secretion, *shen-men,* suprarenal gland, uterus	external genital

Note: Asterisk (*) indicates high effectiveness, with curing rate above 90%.

TABLE 6-5 (cont'd)

Diseases	Primary Acupuncture Points	Secondary Acupuncture Points
secondary testitis	testicle, internal secretion, *shen-men,* suprarenal gland, external genital	hip joint, uterus
premature spermatorrhea	uterus, external genital, testicle, internal secretion, *shen-men*	
prostatitis	prostate, testicle, internal secretion, suprarenal gland, pelvis cavum	
lack of control of bladder	testicle, urethra, dermis, spleen, liver	

TABLE 6-6

Internal Secretion System

Diseases	Acupuncture Points
pituitary dwarfism	kidney, internal secretion, brain point, testicle (male), ovary (female)
mastoplastia	internal secretion, brain point, mammary gland
*swelling of mammary gland	mammary gland, internal secretion, occiput, suprarenal gland
disorder in internal secretion	internal secretion, brain point, dermis, kidney, testicle (male), ovary (female)

TABLE 6-7

Infectious Diseases

Diseases	Primary Acupuncture Points	Secondary Acupuncture Points
*mumps	parotid gland, internal secretion, cheek, dermis	
chicken pox	lung, internal secretion, suprarenal gland, occiput, *shen-men*	
*malaria (prevention)	dermis, internal secretion, suprarenal gland, liver, spleen	
acute & chronic hepatitis	liver, sympathetic, spleen, hepatitis point, liver *yang*	gall, internal secretion
bacterial dysentery	large intestine, small intestine, sympathetic, lung	

Note: Asterisk (*) indicates high effectiveness, with curing rate above 90%.

TABLE 6-8

Surgical Diseases

Diseases	Primary Acupuncture Points	Secondary Acupuncture Points
°strained occiput	neck vertebra, *shen-men*, external genital	
°shoulder periarthritis	shoulder joint, shoulder, *shen-men*, collarbone, suprarenal gland	
°mastitis	mammary gland, internal secretion, suprarenal gland, thorax	
acute & chronic appendicitis	appendix, large intestine, sympathetic, lung	
ascarid in gall	gall, sympathetic, liver, duodenum	
ruptured anus	lower section of rectum, lung, large intestine, spleen	
hemorrhoids	lower section of rectum, large intestine, dermis, spleen, suprarenal gland	
prolapse of anus	lower section of rectum, large intestine, dermis, spleen	
vasculitis	sympathetic, kidney, heart, suprarenal gland, liver, spleen, heat point, corresponding area	internal secretion
frostbite (1-2°)	corresponding area, occiput, spleen, suprarenal gland, lung, heat point	
°furuncle; felon; carbuncle	corresponding area, *shen-men*, occiput, suprarenal gland	
erysipelas	corresponding area, (pricking), occiput, suprarenal gland, internal secretion, lung	*shen-men*
pain relief in bone fracture	corresponding area, *shen-men*, kidney, dermis, suprarenal gland	
°sprain; injury caused by crush	corresponding area, *shen-men*, dermis	heat point

Note: Asterisk (°) indicates high effectiveness, with curing rate above 90%.

TABLE 6-8 (cont'd)

Diseases	Primary Acupuncture Points	Secondary Acupuncture Points
habitual disjoint	corresponding area, supra-renal gland, dermis, spleen, liver	
*acute cellulitis	corresponding area, supra-renal gland, *shen-men*, spleen	

TABLE 6-9

Gynemetrical Diseases

Diseases	Primary Acupuncture Points	Secondary Acupuncture Points
*painful menstruation	uterus, internal secretion, sympathetic, kidney	
leukorrhea	uterus, internal secretion, ovary	
irregular menstruation	uterus, internal secretion, ovary, kidney	
menopause	uterus, internal secretion, ovary, kidney, liver	
inflammation of uterine appendage	ovary, internal secretion, *shen-men*, uterus	
inflammation of uterine lining	uterus, ovary, internal secre-tion, lung, external genital	
chronic inflammation of pelvis cavum	ovary, uterus, internal secretion, pelvis cavum	
*postpartum uteralgia	uterus, sympathetic, *shen-men*, dermis, spleen	
prolapse of uterus	uterus, dermis, sympathetic, external genital	
metrorrhagia	uterus, brain point, internal secretion, liver, spleen, kidney, lung	
external vaginal itching	external genital (pricking), *shen-men*, lung, internal secretion, occiput	suprarenal gland

Note: Asterisk (*) indicates high effectiveness, with curing rate above 90%.

TABLE 6-10

Diseases of the Five Sense Organs

Diseases	Primary Acupuncture Points	Secondary Acupuncture Points
car sickness; sea sickness (prevention)	occiput, stomach, inner ear, *shen-men,* minor occipital nerve	
*furuncle on outer ear	kidney, inner ear, internal secretion, outer ear	
*otitis media	kidney, inner ear, internal secretion, occiput, outer ear	
tinnitus aurium	kidney, occiput, inner ear, outer ear	
lessening hearing power	kidney, occiput, inner ear, outer ear, suprarenal gland	
nose bleeding	inner nose, suprarenal gland, forehead, lung	pressing ear apex
nasovestibular ulcer	inner nose, suprarenal gland, forehead, lung	
*nasosinuitis	inner nose, suprarenal gland, forehead, lung	
allergic rhinitis	inner nose, suprarenal gland, forehead, internal secretion, lung	
hypertrophic rhinitis	inner ear, suprarenal gland, forehead, lung	
hoarseness	throat, heart, lung, *shen-men,* internal secretion	
*uvular edema	throat, *shen-men,* suprarenal gland, lung	
chronic pharyngitis	throat, internal secretion, lung, suprarenal gland	
chronic laryngitis	throat, heart, internal secretion, lung, soft palate	
*acute tonsilitis	tonsil, throat, ear apex blood-letting	
*pain after tonsillectomy	tonsil, throat, *shen-men*	
*Ménière's syndrome	kidney, *shen-men,* occiput, inner ear, dermis	stomach, minor occipital nerve

Note: Asterisk (*) indicates high effectiveness, with curing rate above 90%.

TABLE 6-11

Mouth Diseases

Diseases	Acupuncture Points
obstruction of tooth-cutting	upper jowl, lower jowl, toothache point, soft palate
ulcer in mouth	mouth, internal secretion, *shen-men*, tongue, lung
*nervous toothache	upper jowl, lower jowl, *shen-men*, toothache point, soft palate
loose tooth	kidney, upper jowl, lower jowl, occiput
periodontitis	upper jowl, lower jowl, mouth, suprarenal gland, kidney
glossitis	tongue, mouth, internal secretion, heart, lung

Note: Asterisk (*) indicates high effectiveness, with curing rate above 90%.

TABLE 6-12

Eye Diseases

Diseases	Acupuncture Points
*stye	eye, liver, spleen
*chalazion	eye, liver, spleen
*acute conjunctivitis	eye, liver, lung
eruptive conjunctivitis	eye, liver, suprarenal gland, lung
electric ophthalmia	kidney, liver, eye, *shen-men*
nyctalopia	liver, eye_2, eye, occiput
double vision	kidney, liver, eye_2, eye
astigmatism	kidney, liver, eye, eye_2, occiput
myopia	kidney, liver, eye_2, eye, new eye
chronic glaucoma	kidney, liver, eye_1, eye_2, eye

Note: Asterisk (*) indicates high effectiveness, with curing rate above 90%.

TABLE 6-13

Skin Diseases

Diseases	Acupuncture Points
*inflammation of hair follicle	corresponding area (pricking), lung, occiput, internal secretion, suprarenal gland
shingles	corresponding area (pricking), lung, occiput, internal secretion, suprarenal gland
dermatophiliasis	shen-men, lung, occiput, internal secretion, suprarenal gland, parotid gland
*urticaria	shen-men, lung, occiput, internal secretion, suprarenal gland
verruca simplex	lung, internal secretion, occiput, suprarenal gland, corresponding area (pricking)
neurogentic dermatitis	corresponding area (pricking), lung, occiput, suprarenal gland, parotid gland
dermatitis solaris	shen-men, lung, internal secretion, suprarenal gland
allergic dermatitis	lung, internal secretion, occiput, suprarenal gland, corresponding area (pricking)
prickly heat	lung, suprarenal gland, occiput, shen-men
alopecia areata	corresponding area (pricking), kidney, lung internal secretion
hair loss	kidney, lung, internal secretion, occiput
sebaceous dermatitis	lung, internal secretion, spleen, occiput, suprarenal gland, kidney
rosacea	outer nose (pricking), lung, internal secretion, suprarenal gland
acne	lung, internal secretion, testicle, cheek (pricking)
vitiligo	lung, internal secretion, occiput, suprarenal gland, corresponding area (pricking)
verruca plana	lung, suprarenal gland, occiput, large intestine, corresponding area
eczema	lung, suprarenal gland, occiput, large intestine, corresponding area
diaper rash	corresponding area (pricking), lung, occiput, suprarenal gland
scleroderma	lung, occiput, internal secretion, suprarenal gland, liver, spleen, brain point
sprue	mouth, internal secretion, suprarenal gland, occiput, lung

Note: Asterisk (*) indicates high effectiveness, with curing rate above 90%.

CHAPTER 7

Methods of Ear Acupuncture

The effectiveness of ear acupuncture treatment depends to some extent on the active cooperation between medical personnel and patients. The medical personnel must have the revolutionary spirit to serve the people whole-heartedly, give patients attentive treatment, and relieve their pains. They must patiently explain the merits of ear acupuncture, inspire the active spirit of patients, and convince them to willingly accept the treatment and to cooperate. Of course, the medical personnel must master ear acupuncture techniques in order to give effective treatment. Generally, ear acupuncture techniques and process are stated as follows:

(1) (Examination of pain sensitive point: The accuracy of locating the pain sensitive point is closely related to the efficacy of treatment and is the key to the success of ear acupuncture. Therefore, in treating a patient, we must first make correct diagnosis and then proceed to explore pain sensitive points in corresponding areas. When the probe *(t'an-p'eng)*—if no probe is available, a match stick will do—presses a pain sensitive point, the patient will react with frowning, blinking, crying pain, or dodging. The probe must be handled gently, slowly and smoothly. In a few cases it may not be easy to locate pain sensitive points on the auricle. If so, massage the acupuncture points area a little and then proceed again, or examine the corresponding areas on the other ear. If there is still no reaction at the ear acupuncture points, then stop for a while. If after repeated exploration pain sensitive points are still not

located, then just go ahead to insert needles at proper acupuncture points for specific diseases.

(2) Number of acupuncture points to be needled: Generally, three to five points are best. Either use needles on both ears or just on the one of the troubled side. The duration of treatment depends on specific cases, but usually one series of treatment takes ten times. After an interval of 5-7 days, proceed with the second series of treatment.

(3) The needle must be thoroughly sterilized in order to prevent the auricle from infection. For sterilization, use a cotton ball dipped in 75% alcohol to rub the auricle from inside to outside, from top to bottom, and from anterior to posterior. (After treatment, if the acupuncture point is found to have been infected, it should be rubbed with 2.5% iodine. If necessary, insert needles at acupuncture points such as outer ear, suprarenal gland, occiput, and kidney to counteract infection.)

(4) When inserting the needle, use the left thumb to stabilize the acupuncture point area and the left index finger to support the back side of the acupuncture point. This way the acupuncturist can not only control the depth of the insertion to avoid penetration of the auricle, but also reduce the patient's pain. The needle must be twisted 180° clockwise into the point. It should be done with accuracy and speed.

(5) After insertion, the needle must be left inside, generally, for 20-30 minutes, but for 1-2 hours or longer in cases of chronic diseases. In treating strained joints, during the time when the needle is left in place, it can be twisted once or twice to strengthen the stimulation. At the same time, move the affected joint to reinforce the efficacy of treatment.

(6) Hold a dry cotton ball ready when the needle is being pulled out. If the acupuncture point bleeds, the cotton ball can be used to stop bleeding. According to our clinical experience, the acupuncture points like *shen-men,* occiput, internal secretion, and kidney are easy to bleed, and patients with high blood pressure or blood platelet cytopenia also bleed easily. In inserting the needle, the acupuncturist must take care to avoid small blood vessels. But in our clinical observation, we also discover that

sometimes a few drops of blood actually help improve the efficacy of treatment.

(7) In our clinical experience, it is more effective to use No. 28 rather than No. 30 needle. Sometimes we used several needles in one acupuncture point, and the result was more satisfactory. Generally speaking, in cases of chronic diseases or in cases where other methods are not effective, the use of several needles in one acupuncture point often produces better results.

Rules Against Acupuncture Treatment

Generally, most patients can be treated by ear acupuncture. In very few cases, patients may react with different degrees of dizziness, paleness, cold sweat, unusual low blood pressure, and a similar syndrome.

In the following cases, ear acupuncture should not be used:

(1) During the first five months of pregnancy, a woman should not be treated by ear acupuncture. It is absolutely forbidden to treat pregnant women who are susceptible to miscarriage. After the fifth month of pregnancy, acupuncture points of uterus, ovary, internal secretion, abdomen, and pelvis cavum should not be used in order to prevent miscarriage or pre-mature delivery.

(2) Patients who are over-fatigued, hungry, enfeebled, or have serious cases of anemia should not be treated by ear acupuncture. If ear acupuncture is absolutely necessary, the patient must lie down to avoid acupuncture sickness. When an old patient who suffers arteriolosclerosis and hypertension is inserted with the needle or his lowering pressure trough is treated with bloodletting, he must first rest for half an hour before the treatment and lie down during the treatment. After the treatment, he must be kept under observation for half an hour before being allowed to leave in order to avoid an unpredictable development.

(3) If the auricle suffers frostbite or inflammation, it should not be inserted with an acupuncture needle to prevent spreading of the inflammation. If ear acupuncture is absolutely necessary, then avoid inserting the needle near the inflamed area. Otherwise,

needle the acupuncture points of the outer ear, suprarenal gland, occiput, and kidney to cure frostbite or inflammation first before other diseases are treated.

Treating Acupuncture Sickness

The symptoms of acupuncture sickness are dizziness, fainting spell, paleness, cold sweating, and blood pressure lowering. Treating methods are as follows:

(1) No need to pull out the needle if the acupuncture sickness is slight. The patient can just lie down to rest for a while and drink some warm water. The acupuncturist should talk to the patient to relieve his psychological tension.

(2) If the acupuncture sickness is serious, the needle must be taken out immediately, and the patient's head should be lowered. Then insert needles into the acupuncture points of the suprarenal gland, dermis, heart, and occiput, and the patient will recover.

(3) If after inserting needles, the helix feels particularly painful, or the patient suffers headache, dizziness, nervousness, vomiting, difficulty in opening the mouth, cold lower limbs, or numbness all over the body, such syndromes are usually caused by too deep an insertion into the acupuncture points of the suprarenal gland, sympathetic, and internal secretion. Generally, such syndromes will disappear when the needles are slightly pulled back. If they persist, withdraw the needles and the syndromes will disappear.

Introducing Several Auxiliary Methods

In the development of ear acupuncture skills, we also studied and incorporated experiences of other medical units. Several auxiliary methods of ear acupuncture have been found helpful:

(1) Leaving the needle in place: Use a hypodermic needle, generally available in drug stores. If it is unavailable and has to be made, use No. 28 or No. 30 stainless wire or a cover from an intravenous fluid bottle. It should be made into the shape of a tadpole or a triangular-shaped tack. After the needle is inserted

into the acupuncture point and left inside, it continually provides stimulation. It is particularly appropriate for chronic conditions or for treating patients who are unable to appear for daily treatment.

Method:

a. The auricle should be sterilized as usual.

b. Hold sterilized hypodermic needle or home-made thumb tack with a pair of forceps and insert it into the acupuncture point. The needle end left outside the skin is then fixed firmly with bandage.

c. The needle can be left inside for 7-10 days.

Attention:

a. The patient should be told to press the spot with his finger 2-3 times daily to strengthen stimulation and improve the efficacy of treatment.

b. This method is inappropriate when the weather is warm. It may cause infection of the auricle.

c. As long as the needle is left inside, the auricle should be kept dry while taking a bath or washing the hair.

d. Two or three days after the needle has been left inside, if the auricle appears swollen, it indicates infection. The following steps should be immediately taken:

1. Insert needles into these acupuncture points — outer ear, suprarenal gland, occiput, and kidney.

2. Inject sulfadiazine or penicillin. The amount is to be determined by a doctor.

(2) Ear acupuncture point liquid injection method: (Sometimes called ear acupuncture point drug injection method or ear acupuncture point sealing method). Use appropriate non-irritating liquid medicine and inject it into the ear acupuncture point. This method has the effect not only of ear acupuncture treatment but also of drug cure.

Commonly used medicines: 0.5-1.0% novocain, vitamin B_1, B_{12}, C, placental tissue fluid, placental globulin, liver extract, serum, penicillin, and streptomycin.

Method:

a. The auricle should be sterilized as usual.

b. Select liquid medicine and ear acupuncture point in accordance with the disease.

c. Each acupuncture point should be injected 0.2-0.4 cc. It should be injected between cartilage and dermis to form a small lump.

d. Inject once every two or three days, each treatment consisting of 5-7 injections.

Attention:

a. Attention should be paid to maintaining aseptic conditions to prevent infection.

b. Strictly forbid injection of irritating liquid medicine which may destroy tissue.

(3) Ear acupuncture point cutting treatment: This method produces stronger stimulation at ear acupuncture point, suitable for chronic conditions and persistent diseases.

Method:

a. The auricle should be sterilized as usual.

b. Cut open about 0.2 cm. the ear acupuncture point with sterilized surgical knife tip and let a few drops of blood. Then apply first-aid cream and wrap it up. Cut 2-4 points each time.

c. Cut once every 7-10 days, each treatment consisting of three cuts.

Attention:

a. Thorough sterilization to prevent infection.

b. Strictly forbid taking a bath or washing the hair within three to five days after cutting to prevent infection.

c. The opening should not be too big or too deep. If the method is found ineffective after three cuts, try other methods.

(4) Ear acupuncture point pricking treatment: This method produces stronger stimulation at ear acupuncture point. It is recommended for treating chronic conditions and persistent diseases.

Method:

a. The auricle should be sterilized as usual.

b. Insert sterilized triple-edged needle into acupuncture point to reach cartilage beneath skin and then prick it up. Two to four points each time.

c. Apply antibiotic cream to the pricked points and then wrap them up.

d. Prick once every 3-5 days, each treatment consisting of three prickings.

Attention:

a. The edge of the triple-edged needle should not be too sharp. The principle is that the skin should not be torn when it is pricked.

b. Strictly forbid taking a bath and washing the hair to prevent infection.

(5) Ear acupuncture point electric stimulation treatment: Connect the needle with commonly used electric-therapy machine and insert it into acupuncture point. This way the electric current will continually stimulate the acupuncture point to effect a cure. This method is to be used in chronic conditions or in cases where regular needle insertion is less effective.

Method:

a. When both ears are inserted with needles, the two needles are attached to positive and negative electrodes. The electric circuit should be on for 10-15 minutes and the volume is determined by the patient who should feel a slight sensation of burning at the ear acupuncture points.

When only one ear is inserted with needles, they are attached to one electrode and the patient's hand holds the other. The volume of electricity is determined in the same manner as above.

b. When no needle is available, a probe attached to one electrode can be used to press upon the acupuncture point and the patient holds the other. The volume of electricity is determined in the same manner as above, and the treatment should last for 2-3 minutes.

The above method is applied once every other day, each treatment consisting of 7-10 insertions.

(6) Ear acupuncture point massage method: The method is to massage or press upon ear acupuncture points in the following manner:

a. Pressing points with a probe.

Use a probe to press lightly and rub ear acupuncture points. Each treatment lasts for 2-3 minutes.

b. Pressing points with rapeseeds.

Place rapeseeds on ear acupuncture points, and hold them with bandage.

c. Pressing points with match stick.

Place 0.1–0.2 cm. match sticks on ear acupuncture points and hold them with a bandage.

When methods *b* and *c* are used, the patient is told to rub the treated spots three times each day and to remove rapeseeds or match sticks after seven days. This method is suitable for treating old men and young children.

CHAPTER 8

Techniques in Applying the Acupuncture Needle

In the chapter "Plain Dialogue: Treatise on Basic Principles of Needle Insertion" of *The Yellow Emperor's Classic of Internal Medicine,* acupuncture techniques are discussed. "Diseases may be divided into benign and malignant types, and the needle may be inserted shallowly or deeply. Each method has its merits, and none should be used in extreme." This plain dialectical thought of the ancients has remained influential in clinical treatment of diseases down the centuries. The ear acupuncture treatment not only has retained and incorporated skills common in acupuncture and moxibustion such as pricking, insertion, massage, and leaving the needle in place, but also has developed specific techniques because of the unique characteristics of the auricle. Furthermore, since one patient is different from another, some diseases often show different symptoms, and different diseases sometimes show the same symptom. Therefore, different techniques of needle insertion should be used for different patients. We ought to apply the needle with flexibility and to try a variety of techniques. Only this way needle insertion will fully regulate organs, promote circulation of air and blood, and quickly turn troubled conditions to recovery.

After a great deal of clinical applications, we come to the conclusion that in order for ear acupuncture techniques to be effective, attention should be paid to four factors: accuracy of acupuncture points, correct direction, speed of insertion, and depth of insertion.

Accuracy of Acupuncture Points

The area of the auricle is very small, and acupuncture points are concentrated. Whether acupuncture points can be correctly located largely determines the curing effect. For example, in treating sciatic neuritis, satisfactory result can be achieved after 4-10 times of treatment. In our unit, however, one medic treated a poor peasant woman's sciatic neuritis continually 20 times without satisfactory results. The pain was slightly relieved but the disease not cured. A sense of heaviness in the hips and lower limbs was never reduced. After repeated check-ups, we did not discover any problem in our diagnosis and selection of acupuncture points. Further study revealed that the problem was a matter of accuracy. The medic missed the major acupuncture point "sciatic nerve" in the combination of points used for treating sciatic neuritis and instead inserted the needle into "constipation," a nearby point. Later, when we inserted the needle into the correct acupuncture point, the patient immediately felt relief all over her body, the pain deadened, and the sense of heaviness in the hips and lower limbs greatly reduced.

Accuracy in locating acupuncture points is the prerequisite to curing diseases. Therefore, in our clinical work we treat a patient in his first visit with great care. On the basis of correct diagnosis, all acupuncture points to be inserted are ascertained by means of a probe or an ear acupuncture points locating device.

Correct Direction

In the past we were dubious about the question of direction of needle insertion. We felt that the auricle is so small that any talk about direction of needle insertion was mystifying. As long as the needle was inserted into the correct acupuncture point and stayed there firmly, that was enough. Actually, this attitude suggests bias and blindness. In clinical treatment we came across conditions such as this: in cases of obstruction in movement or of acute painful conditions, if reaction to needle insertion is insufficient, the needle can be withdrawn slightly (but not out of the skin), and then it is inserted in a different direction. Usually, the patient will react differently. For example, in treating a patient with pain on his right upper arm, we located the pain sensitive point at his auricle. When the needle was inserted into this point, the patient reacted fairly strongly and his pain was reduced. But his right upper arm still could not be lifted and could be moved outward only with difficulty. When we changed the direction of the insertion, the troubled arm could be lifted up. When we changed its direction for the second time, the arm could be moved outward. After continually changing the direction of insertion three times, the patient could move his right arm freely.

The angle and direction of needle insertion are related to different locations of ear acupuncture points. Different point locations determine different angles and directions of needle insertion. Because the auricle has concaves and convexes and is folded and curved at places without definite direction and angle, it is difficult to accurately insert the needle into the correct point. For instance, the needle is inserted at a 90° angle vertically into the acupuncture points of the heart, lung, spleen, stomach, kidney, bladder, small intestine, and large intestine in cavum concha, and cymba concha. It is called straight insertion. The needle is inserted at 45°-60° angle into the acupuncture points of the shoulder, wrist, elbow, finger, toe, sciatic nerve, and constipation in scaphoid fossa, antitragus, anthelix, upper and lower crura of anthelix. It is called slant insertion. Again, inserting the needle into the "dermis" point in a slanting direction has a tranquilizing effect while in a straight line it has the effect of excitement. This means that the same acupuncture point may produce different effects when the directions of needle insertion are different. Therefore, in clinical application different directions of needle insertion are necessary for treating different diseases when the same acupuncture point is used. For instance, the "heart" point is inserted at a 90° angle in a straightforward direction for treating common cardiovascular diseases, but it is inserted at a slant angle of 45° for treating pericarditis. This has been verified in clinical practices.

Our tentative conclusion is that correct direction is an important aspect of accuracy of acupuncture point location. Therefore, whether a direction is correct or not is really an extension or implementation of whether an acupuncture point is accurate or not. It is an important aspect of ear acupuncture technique which should not be overlooked.

Speed of Insertion

Chairman Mao once said: "Contradiction and struggle are universal and absolute phenomena, but methods to solve contradiction, viz., forms of struggle, differ according to the nature of contradiction." Speedy and slow paces of inserting the needle are the two aspects of the contradiction. In ear acupuncture speedy needle insertion is stressed because of the particular contradiction in ear acupuncture treatment.

We all know that the auricle is an irregular cartilage tissue structure, different from any other part of the human body. The cartilage tissue has dense structure, tightly attached to the skin, with rich nerve endings and blood vessels. Then, needle inserting locations are situated at pain sensitive points. Therefore, compared with other types of acupuncture and moxibustion, intramuscular and intravenous injections, it is more painful. "Different contradictions can be solved only by different methods." Because of the peculiar nature of ear acupuncture, a speedy or slow pace of needle insertion not only causes different sensation and reaction but also produces a different curing effect. We repeatedly verified this point through inserting "experimental needles" in ourselves and in treating workers, peasants, and soldiers. Speedy needle insertion will not only reduce pain but help in getting active cooperation of patients.

Under usual circumstances, the needle must be inserted rapidly, but this rule is by no means absolute. For instance, in treating certain diseases, if the method requires increasing stimulation or a strengthening twist, then the insertion can be deliberately slowed down.

Depth of Insertion

Generally speaking, needle insertion must produce a definite volume of stimulation or the effect of treatment will not be as good. Clinical experience tells us that grasp of proper volume of stimulation and skill in applying the needle greatly affect efficacy of treatment. "External causes are the condition of change." "In a suitable temperature an egg hatches into a chicken." For a patient with tuberculosis, for instance, without using sufficient antibiotics in treatment, he cannot be cured. This principle in using medicine applies to acupuncture. In using medicine, the quantity is determined on the basis of the severity of disease; in inserting the needle, strong or weak stimulation depends on different cases. We know that the volume of stimulation is realized to a great extent by the depth of insertion; "depth" is the means and "volume" the end. A certain degree of depth produces a certain volume of stimulation. For instance, for patient of spermatorrhea, shallow or deep needle insertion produces different curing effects. Our study of numerous clinical cases proves that in treating parenchymatous diseases, fevers, acute pains, and inflammations, deep needle insertion produces better results and shortens the period of treatment. On the other hand, in treating deficiency diseases, chills, and chronic diseases such as chronic anemia and cardiasthenia, only shallow needle insertion with prolonged treatment will produce the expected result. The term "depth" used here is of course relative to the term "shallow." Our understanding is that for some diseases deep insertion is better than shallow insertion, but it does not mean the deeper the better. Insertion should be deep enough to penetrate the cartilage but not so deep as to penetrate the skin on the opposite side. By the same token, shallow insertion does not mean the shallower the better. Mere penetration of the skin with the needle hanging shakily on the auricle will not produce a curing effect. The needle must be inserted into the cartilage and stay firmly in a definite angle. What is called deep insertion and shallow insertion in ear acupuncture are similar to that in regular acupuncture but with some difference.

If in inserting the needle one follows the rules of determining the accurate acupuncture point and correct direction, speedy insertion, and deep insertion, the patient will feel strong sensations. Concretely stated, the patient's auricle will feel the sensations of heaviness, burning, warmth, coolness, or jumping. Then, a satisfactory curing effect will result.

In addition, we shall discuss briefly our experience in twisting the needle during and after its insertion and other related problems.

The Question of Twisting the Needle During and After Its Insertion: Generally, when the needle is being twisted, it can be twisted at a 180° turn. After the insertion, the needle is not moved in and out or twisted; only in cases where the insertion fails to produce an effect, it is moved in and out or twisted once or twice.

The Question of Using Thick or Thin Needle: The needle size is determined by different diseases which require different volumes of stimulation. Generally speaking, a thick needle is used for diseases (such as acute diseases) which require strong stimulation; otherwise, a thin needle is used. Take vasculitis treatment for example. The combination of acupuncture points we commonly use is the heart, liver, sympathetic, corresponding area, dermis, internal secretion, and suprarenal gland. For the first five acupuncture points, we use a thick needle, viz., 0.5 dm. long No. 28; for the last two acupuncture points, a thin needle, viz., 0.5 dm. long No. 30 is used. In order to increase the volume of stimulation, sometimes we can use several needles in one acupuncture point, that is, inserting two or three needles in one point.

The Question of Leaving the Needle in Place: We consider this method supplementary to the "deep" method for the purpose of increasing "volume of stimulation." The duration of time for the needle to stay in place is determined by the disease condition. Generally speaking, one hour is best. For some patients of chronic diseases, leaving the needle in place for 2-3 hours will produce better results. For children the duration can be shorter, or the method is not used at all.

CHAPTER 9

Diagnosis by
Examining the Auricle

Through numerous clinical observations, we discover that when a certain internal organ or a certain part of the human body suffers an ailment, especially organic disease, in most cases the corresponding part or specific area of the auricle will show a *yang* (positive) reaction. The pathological development is reflected in skin discoloration, deformation, peeling, and appearance of papules. For instance, most patients of gastric ulcer will have a small, round-shaped point at the stomach acupuncture point area of the auricle, a pathological reaction distinguishable from the normal skin around it. Many patients who have undergone gastrectomy will have a thin, dull-red or white crescent-shaped scar at the stomach area of the auricle.

Chairman Mao teaches us, "It is necessary to build up a system of concepts and theories by subjecting the abundant perceptual data to a process of remolding and reconstructing—discarding the crude and selecting the refined, eliminating the false and retaining the true, proceeding from one point to another, and going through the outside into the inside." We carefully studied and analyzed the accumulated data from examining more than 20,000 patients and reached some tentative conclusions concerning pathological phenomena shown at the auricle, such as those of gastric diseases, pulmonary diseases, chronic and acute appendicitis, hepatitis, furuncles, gynecological diseases, and some skin diseases. This knowledge provides useful reference for supportive diagnosis and differential diagnosis. Auricle examination diagnosis is particularly useful in mountain areas, countrysides, and clinics with inadequate medical facilities. It has practical significance in promoting works of preventive medicine and treatment among the masses and fits well Chairman Mao's strategy of "grasping revolution, promoting production and other work, and preparedness against war."

Methods of Examination

(1) When examining the ear, use thumb and index finger to stretch the auricle and examine the anatomical features, step by step, from top to bottom, and from outside to inside.

(2) When a *yang* reaction is spotted, use the index finger to prop up the auricular posterior in order to stretch the skin for accurate identification of the *yang* reaction.

(3) When the *yang* reactions are found to be different at the two auricles, comparison and contrast must be made and the location, nature, and scope of the pathological reaction analyzed in order to reach preliminary diagnosis.

(4) If a swollen or tubercular reaction is discovered, use a finger or a probe to test the size and hardness of the tubercle, its mobility, the regularity of its edge, and its pain sensitivity.

(5) When examining triangular fossa and cymba concha, use a probe or a match stick to stretch out the crus of helix to expose the area.

Reactions of Common Diseases at the Auricle

TABLE 9-1

Auricular Reactions and Disease Classification

Classification of Reactions	Symptoms	Common Diseases
discoloration	(1) point-shaped or flake-shaped white, red, or opaque grey (2) white point with red rim	chronic and acute gastritis, gastro-duodenal ulcer, chronic and acute tracheitis, hepatobiliary disease, nephritis, all kinds of arthritis, headache, dizziness, acute appendicitis, eye diseases, gynecological diseases, change of blood pressure, heart diseases
deformation	(1) point-shaped depression (2) rope-shaped or tubercular pro-tuberance	tuberculosis, chronic appendicitis, hepatomegalia, swelling, heart diseases, metaplastic ossification, crippling caused by external injury, hypertrophy, deformation, or degeneration of vertebra
papules	red or white pointed papules (like goose-flesh)	gynecological diseases, large and small intestinal diseases, kidney diseases, cystitis, heart diseases, tuberculosis, acute and chronic bronchitis
skin peeling	white flaky, husk-like surface at the lung area and lower rim of crus of helix	all kinds of skin diseases, gyneco-logical diseases, malfunction of absorption and vicarious function, constipation

TABLE 9-2

Auricular Pathological Reactions of Common Diseases

Disease	Location	Reactions
acute gastritis	stomach area	red, shiny point or flake
chronic gastritis	stomach area	white flake without clear-cut rim, with part of the skin thickened (usually found in hypertrophic gastritis)
sudden onset of chronic gastritis	stomach area	(1) white flake or point with red, shiny rim (2) red or bloodshot point or flake
gastroptosis	stomach area	white flake-shaped swelling without clear-cut rim at the periphery of stomach area near anthelix

TABLE 9-2 (cont'd)
Auricular Pathological Reactions of Common Diseases

Disease	Location	Reactions
gastric ulcer	stomach area	(1) white point with clear-cut rim (2) white or opaque grey with red rim, usually shiny (see plate 9-1)
duodenal ulcer	duodenum	same as above
chronic enteritis	large and small intestine area	bloodshot flake or papule, full of fat
constipation	large and small intestine area	white flake or husky skin peeling, opaque
acute appendicitis	appendix area	bloodshot point or papule
chronic appendicitis	appendix area	often pointed depression or swelling, occasionally white or opaque grey
sudden onset of chronic appendicitis	appendix area	white point with red rim or red flake
acute hepatitis	liver area	(1) red flake or point (2) white center with red rim, usually shiny
hepatomegalia	liver area	white flake-shaped swelling (like half kernel of watermelon seed) with clear-cut rim (right hepatomegalia if at right ear; left hepatomegalia if at left ear). (see plate 9-1)
splenomegalia	spleen area	white flake with red rim, occasionally swelling
tuberculosis — active stage	lung area	bloodshot point or papule, shiny, occasionally oozing blood when rubbed (the same side lung if it appears at the lower side; the opposite side lung if it appears at the upper side)
tuberculosis — calcifying stage	lung area	one or several needle-point depressions
acute pneumonia	between two lungs	red point or papule, sometimes white point with red shiny rim
acute tracheitis	trachea	red point or papule, sometimes white point with red shiny rim
chronic tracheitis	trachea	white point or flake with clear-cut rim, sometimes white papule, but always opaque
sudden onset of chronic tracheitis	trachea	white point or flake or papule, with red rim, always shiny

TABLE 9-2 (cont'd)
Auricular Pathological Reactions of Common Diseases

Disease	Location	Reactions
pulmonary emphysema	lung area	white flake or flake formed by dense points, without clear-cut rim, shiny during onset
excessive dreams, insomnia, irregular heart rhythm, premature contraction	heart area	wrinkled circle with shiny center, occasionally white center
rheumatic heart disease	heart area	white flake without clear-cut rim, occasionally shiny
all kinds of headaches, dizziness	brain point, brain stem, forehead, dermis	red point or white point with red rim, usually shiny
high blood pressure	brain point, brain stem, forehead, dermis	reactions in these areas are the same as in cases of headaches and dizziness; in addition, when suprarenal gland shows red point or flake, heart area shows wrinkled circle, and upper 1/3 of lowering pressure trough shows white point or with red rim, blood pressure is about 150; when middle 1/3 of lowering pressure trough shows reaction, blood pressure is about 200
low blood pressure	brain point, brain stem, forehead, dermis	reactions at head area acupuncture points are the same as in high blood pressure; suprarenal gland has no reaction; when lower 1/3 of lowering pressure trough shows white point or with red rim, it means low blood pressure
acute strained joint	corresponding area	red point or flake
protracted arthritis	corresponding area	white point or flake
sudden onset of chronic arthritis	corresponding area	white point with red rim, always shiny
deformation of spinal column or hypertrophic fracture	corresponding area	rope-shaped, or furuncle type swelling, sometimes rope-shaped depression, either vertical or horizontal
hemorrhoidal tubercle	hemorrhoidal tubercle point, lower end of rectum	white point or flake with red rim, occasionally opaque grey point or flake

TABLE 9-2 (cont'd)

Auricular Pathological Reactions of Common Diseases

Disease	Location	Reactions
ruptured anus	hemorrhoidal tubercle point, anus	white point with red saw-edged rim, occasionally, red point in radiating shape
benign tumor	corresponding area	swelling abscess underneath skin, movable, with clear-cut rim, not painful when pressed (not many cases reported, further research needed)
malignant tumor	corresponding area	(1) cartilaginous protuberance, with no clear-cut rim, unmovable (2) sometimes white or opaque grey flake, pain sensitive (not many cases reported, futher research needed)
painful menstruation	uterus area	white or red point, with fat
profuse menstruation and leukorrhea	uterus area	bloodshot, pointed papule (see plate 9-2)
scanty menstruation or short-term menopause	uterus area	white point or flake, opaque, occasionally, husky skin-peeling
neurogenic dermatitis	corresponding part of lung area	husky skin-peeling, difficult to rub off (see plate 9-2)
chronic urticaria	corresponding part of lung area	same as above
eczema	corresponding part of lung area	husky skin-peeling, difficult to rub off
sebaceous dermatitis	entire auricle	same as above, with fat
scale-shaped dermatitis	entire auricle	scale-shaped layer, dry and opaque
obstruction in absorptive function	entire auricle	dry and skin-peeling, opaque
post-surgery	corresponding area	white shallow line or crescent scar, occasionally dark grey
using internal contraceptive medicine	uterus, cymba concha, cavum concha, internal secretion	white flake-shaped skin-peeling, like the top layer of lichen

Dialectic Diagnosis in Auricular Examination

In auricular examination, attention must be paid to the unique characteristics of "several reactions of one disease" and of "several pathological reactions at one acupuncture point."

(1) Red or bloodshot point and flake, sometimes with red rim, or red papule, with fat and shiny color, are symptoms of acute inflammatory diseases.

(2) White point or flake, depression, swelling, and white papule, always without fat and shiny color, are symptoms of chronic organic diseases.

(3) Tubercle-shaped swelling or point and opaque grey flake are usually symptoms of tumors.

(4) Husky skin-peeling (difficult to rub off) is often seen in all kinds of skin diseases or obstruction in absorptive and vicarious functions.

(5) Lineal, round, or crescent white or opaque grey scars are often shown after surgery or external injury.

The above shows that auricular pathological reactions follow general patterns. If in examining auricular reactions we can grasp the specific and general rules and the unique characteristics of "several reactions of one disease" and "several pathological reactions at one acupuncture point," and compare with the patient's symptoms, we can attain preliminary "dialectic diagnosis."

For example, pharyngitis and tonsillitis both have reactions at a particular point (tonsil$_4$). The specific reaction of pharyngitis is several white or red points without clear-cut rim; the specific reaction of tonsillitis is red or bloodshot flake with clear-cut rim. The two inflammatory diseases often show different reactions at the tonsil acupuncture point.

Attention in Auricular Examination

(1) Close attention must be paid to different conditions of skin in winter and summer, in old patients and children, and of individual's body difference.

(2) Do not rub, wash, and stretch the auricle before examina-

tion so that the skin will not change color, the *yang* reaction will not be rubbed off, and the accuracy of diagnosis will not be affected. If the depressed area of the auricle is not clean, use a cotton ball to gently wipe it toward one direction.

(3) When a *yang* reaction is discovered, consult traditional Chinese visceral theory so as to make a comprehensive dialectic analysis to reach diagnosis.

(4) On the auricle of a healthy person often can be found some phenomena (such as deep color, white tubercle, small pimple, or scar of frostbite). Such are "pseudo-symptoms." The method of differentiation is: first observe, then press it. If no pain is felt when pressed, the phenomenon is a pseudo-*yang* reaction.

(5) There must be sufficient light. Natural light is best, but at night a flashlight can be used for penetrating examination.

Some Insights in Auricular Examination and Diagnosis

Chairman Mao teaches us: "The viewpoint of practice is the first and basic viewpoint in the theory of knowledge of dialectical materialism." From ear acupuncture treatment to auricular examination and diagnosis, we went through repeated tests and step by step experiments. We have reached the following tentative conclusions throughout our practice:

(1) Through auricular examination and diagnosis, we have further confirmed the definite locations of ear acupuncture points. For instance, pathological reactions of paralysis, metaplastic osteosis of the spinal column, prolapse of lumbar vertebra are shown at the apex of anthelix rather than at the hidden side of anthelix. Again, lungs are divided into upper and lower lungs at cavum concha. The lower lung represents the lung on the same side while the upper lung that on the opposite side.

(2) Through auricular examination and diagnosis, the efficacy of ear acupuncture treatment is improved. It is more effective to insert the needle into pathological reaction points.

(3) Through auricular examination and diagnosis, we have gained further understanding of the visceral theory of traditional Chinese medicine. For instance, the heart controls spirit and will,

thus excessive dreams, insomnia, diseases of the nervous and mental systems are shown in the heart area. Spleen is intimately related to stomach, so chronic gastritis, gastric or duodenal ulcer, and indigestion (obstruction in circulation and digestion) are shown both in the spleen as well as stomach area. Lungs control skin and hair, and thus all skin diseases are shown in the lung area. All these are in agreement with the visceral theory in traditional Chinese medicine.

(4) Auricular examination and diagnosis has opened a new avenue in preliminary diagnosis and differential diagnosis of tumor and acute appendicitis that must be further explored.

The above suggests some of our comprehension of auricular examination and diagnosis in clinical practice. Although we can make accurate diagnosis of some diseases, we know only pathological development in corresponding areas in most cases. Therefore, in clinical application we cannot totally rely on ear examination to reach conclusions but must make specific analysis on the basis of actual conditions.

In short, auricular examination and diagnosis is a new development. Many problems still exist and must be resolved through continual explorations.

CHAPTER 10

A Brief Description of Ear Acupuncture Point Locating Devices and Their Application

Introduction

In previous chapters it is stated that insertion of the needle at pain sensitive points of the auricle can cure diseases. If a pain sensitive point is located in a certain area, does that mean in a particular part of the body? This question interests many people.

For instance, a certain hospital accepted a patient with an acute abdominal ailment, and after physical examination and laboratory tests, the preliminary diagnosis was acute appendicitis. Afterwards, a match stick was used to locate the pain sensitive point only to find that the appendix acupuncture point showed no obvious pain sensitive reaction. On the other hand, the patient's ureter area was clearly pain sensitive. After X-ray examination, urinary lithiasis was confirmed. This case reflects the function of ear acupuncture diagnosis and deserves our further exploration.

The use of a probe (or a match stick) to locate the pain sensitive point for the purpose of differential diagnosis has definite referral value. This is a comparatively simple method, and it depends on the sensitive reaction of the patient during application.

Sometimes, it is difficult to distinguish a genuine from a false pain sensitive point.

Since the successful construction of a vessel and meridian locating device, the medical personnel in Peking, Shanghai, Nanking, and Sian designed a number of small crystalline tube ear acupuncture point locating devices upon the principle that the pain sensitive point is low in electric resistance and high in conductivity. Compared to the probe, the instrument is easy to handle and more accurate. It is a step forward in locating ear acupuncture points.

When we started to use the crystalline tube ear acupuncture point locating device, we discovered that sensitive point exists in the kidney area among 80% of females. At first we thought that the sensitive point in the kidney area meant a kidney ailment. But their urine test showed a *yin* (negative) reaction. What could be the problem?

Then we studied Chairman Mao's teaching, "All genuine knowledge originates in direct experience." Carrying with us ear acupuncture point locating devices, we went to do experiments and tests with patients in the army, villages, factories, and hospitals. We conducted experiments with tens of thousands of patients to determine the interrelationship between a variety of diseases and reactions at ear acupuncture points and reached some preliminary conclusions. For instance, most diseases would be shown at more than 2-5 pain sensitive points on the auricle. Most of the auricular pain sensitive points are valuable for analyzing diseases in corresponding areas. Some diseases have specific auricular pain sensitive points. In a few cases, although patients have some organic disease, no pain sensitive point can be found in the corresponding area of the auricle. These phenomena enhance our understanding of auricular pain sensitive points and enrich and further the clinical significance of ear acupuncture points. At the same time, we discovered some new acupuncture points highly valuable in diagnosis and treatment. Thus we introduced the ear acupuncture point locating device to clinical diagnosis.

The history of clinical use of the ear acupuncture point locat-

ing device is very short, and a more relentless and thorough study
is required for understanding and mastering its potential. Theoretical research concerning the appearance of pain sensitive points or
technicality of the instrument must be further explored through
study and application.

Brief Discussion of Construction of Ear
Acupuncture Point Locating Devices

At present there are many types of ear acupuncture point
locating devices designed upon the theory of electric resistance
at auricular sensitive points. They can be classified into three
general types:

(1) Electric meter: This instrument differentiates the pain
sensitive point from the normal acupuncture point when its meter
shows varying electric currents. Its merit is that its meter directly
points out the current intensity at the pain sensitive point. This
instrument is particularly useful in laboratories. It is expensive
and inconvenient if used by one person who has to examine ear
acupuncture points and read the meter at the same time.

(2) Acoustic indicator: This device uses sound transmitted
through an earphone or microphone to differentiate a pain sensitive point from a normal ear acupuncture point. It is a simple
device, easy to make and low in cost. Its defect is that there is no
clear standard to distinguish one sound from another.

(3) Neon detector: Whether the neon bulb shines or not
differentiates a pain sensitive point from a normal acupuncture
point. Since a neon bulb requires higher glow discharge, the
instrument needs higher electric pressure (about several dozen
volts). As a result, it takes a more powerful battery. This instrument may burn the skin of the ear sometimes, so the patient may
not be receptive to it.

A kind of simple acoustic crystalline tube ear acupuncture
point locating instrument is introduced in the following pages as
reference for experimental construction. The schematic diagram
of the circuit is shown in Figure 10-1.

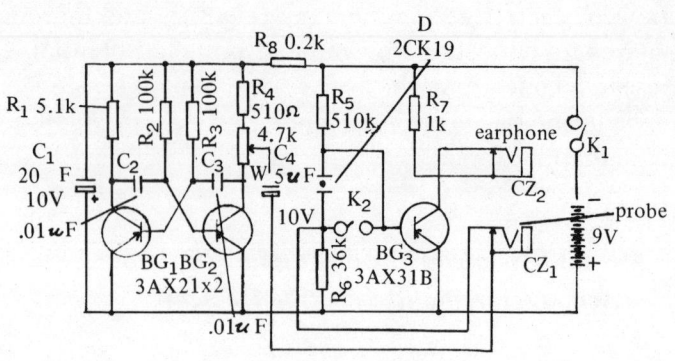

FIGURE 10-1

In the diagram, BG_1, BG_2, R_1, R_2, R_3, R_4, W, C_2 and C_3 together form an automatic multivibrator to produce a signal with a frequency of 1000 hertz, a rectangular pulsating wave, and a pulsatory amplitude of 9 volts. It is transmitted through the potentiometer W and the coupling condenser C_4 as an input signal to pass the body. The potentiometer W can be used to regulate the strength of the signal and thus to control the sensitivity of the instrument.

BG_3 is an audio-frequency amplifier. When the input signal passes through the patient's body and voltage divider R_6, the electric pressure of the signal on both ends of the voltage divider R_6 is coupled at diode D and then amplified at base BG_3. The amplified electric signal passes the earphone to become a sound signal. Here the selection of diode D and its connection method have specific significance.

The diode is connected in such a way that the signal that passes the diode to reach BG_3 must be negative to the electric potential at base BG_3 so as to form a switch.

The diode must be a silica diode with a small reverse current (smaller than 1 microampere), so as to reduce noise in the earphone to such an extent that sound is heard only when the pain sensitive point is located.

The triodes BG_1 and BG_2 should be identical and β should not be lower than 40.

BG_3 is an amplifier tube, so its β ought to be higher (higher than 60), and the resistance of the earphone is about 1500 ohms. The electric current of the collector in BG_1 and BG_2 should be regulated to the level of 1.8 milliampere and that of the collector in BG_3 at the level of 1 milliampere, and the electric current at the base must be lower than 50 microampere when no signal passes through. If an oscillograph is used, attach the Y axis input to the probe and the other electrode to the ground wire of the oscillograph to examine the output signal of the multivibrator. The pulsatory signal must be symmetric, and the wave crest should not be distorted. The current frequency should be 1,000 cycles per second.

Furthermore, K_2 remains open when the instrument is being used. If the pain sensitive point cannot be located, K_2 can be closed. In that case, the earphone keeps transmitting sound, and the pain sensitive point can be recognized by distinguishing the volume of the sound.

This instrument can be set in a transistor box and is small and easy to carry. The earphone can be made a separate part and connected only during use.

Application of the Ear Acupuncture
Point Locating Device

(1) When the instrument is turned on, the earphone (or microphone) will transmit sound (about 1,000 hz). Insert the plug of the probe into the instrument; if no sound is heard in the earphone, it means the instrument is normal.

(2) The acupuncturist holds the probe (that is an electrode) and presses the other electrode at the inner gate acupuncture point (*nan-kuan hsueh*)—better still to fix it with the belt of an electrocardiograph. Then he moves the probe to the patient's seal valley acupuncture point (*ho-kuo hsueh*) or the spinal cord acupuncture point at his auricle and adjusts the electric potential sensitivity of the instrument to allow the earphone to transmit sound. While the acupuncturist determines the sound level, he must keep it in mind. When the probe locates a point with a similar

sound, it is a sensitive point. The acupuncture point without sound suggests a *yin* reaction. The acupuncture point with sound and pricking pain suggests a strong *yang* reaction.

(3) Use the following symbols to record various reactions of each pain sensitive point. Take the kidney point for example:

Kidney   It records the acupuncture point without symbol, showing sound.

Kidney   It records sound and pricking pain, showing a strong *yang* reaction.

Kidney°   It shows a low sound.

Kidney   It means no sound, but shows a pain reaction.

(4) There are two methods to locate pain sensitive points:

a. Examine the auricle from top down, generally, first examine viscera, then body, and finally the four limbs (that is, examine first cavum concha, cymba concha, and triangular fossa, and then anthelix, helix, lobule, scaphoid fossa, and auricular posterior). The symptoms reported by the patient must be checked carefully by examining corresponding areas of the auricle.

b. Use systematic examination. This method requires a good knowledge of the instrument user about reaction patterns of diseases at ear acupuncture points. When the probe locates a pain sensitive point, the entire corresponding area, which is related to the point or may cause the disease, must be fully examined. If the finding fits the symptoms of the disease to form a preliminary diagnosis, then proceed with further examination.

For example, when we were examining a patient, we discovered the gall area show strong *yang* reaction (**gall**). Then we examined three other acupuncture points—liver, shoulder joint, and outer abdomen. If these three points were all pain sensitive, the patient might suffer inflammation of the gall bladder. If the three points were not pain sensitive or only the liver area showed low sound reaction (liver°), then the patient's pain sensitive point at the gall area might be caused by a liver disease. We could exclude the possibility of gall bladder inflammation, and proceed to examine acupuncture points related to diseases of the liver system. This method is suitable for differential diagnosis.

(5) Instrument manipulation skills. The variation of ear acu-

puncture point sensitivity depends on age, sex, working conditions, type and degree of disease, climate, environment, temperature, and humidity. It can also be influenced by the efficiency of the instrument and the acupuncturist's manipulation skills.

The efficiency of the instrument depends on its design and manufacture. As for manipulation skills, we believe that in examining cymba concha, cavum concha, lobule, triangular fossa, and scaphoid fossa where skin is softer, the probe must be handled gently. In examining anthelix and antitragus, the probe can be pressed harder. In distinguishing ear acupuncture points in the same area, the probe must be handled in a consistent manner.

(6) After the instrument is used, remove the probe and earphone and switch it off.

(7) The level of electric pressure of the battery affects the sensitivity of the instrument. Generally, use a 9-volt battery; when the electric pressure is lower than 8 volts, it is no longer useful.

Overall Analysis of the Results of Ear Acupuncture Point Sensitivity Exploration

In the process of examining ear acupuncture point sensitivity, we discovered that a certain disease may have several pain sensitive points or the same sensitive point may appear in a number of diseases. Their interrelationship is rather intricate. If we follow Chairman Mao's teaching, "Correct judgment results from complete and necessary research and from reasoning based on research data," relate identified ear acupuncture pain sensitive points with the pathological history of the patient, and proceed with generalization and analysis, we can reach rather accurate judgment of disease differentiation. An overall generalization and analysis of pain sensitive points identified by an ear acupuncture locating device is an important link in using ear acupuncture points for disease diagnosis. If we cannot make correct analysis, we may make serious error. Even the best instrument will be of no avail.

There are three sources of information for analysis:

(1) The viscera theory of traditional Chinese medicine is a theory of physiological function of the body, pathological develop-

ment, and their interrelationship. In the examination of an ear acupuncture point, the viscera theory can be used to explain the appearance of pain sensitive points, to generalize and analyze pain sensitive points, and to assist in therapeutical treatment as valuable reference.

For example, in a case of fractured bones, aside from the appearance of the pain sensitive point at the auricular corresponding area, usually a pain sensitive point also appears at the kidney area of the auricle, according to the "kidneys control bone" rule in traditional Chinese medicine (see case no. 1). If lungs have organic pathological development, aside from the appearance of the pain sensitive point at the auricular lung area, usually a pain sensitive point also appears at the large intestine area of the auricle, according the rule "lungs and large intestine are intimately related." Again, when pain sensitive points are located at the acupuncture points of the heart, **shen-men,** and dermis, consideration must be given to the possibility that for a patient of heart disease, aside from the appearance of the pain sensitive point at the auricular heart area, it also appears at the small intestine point. If no pain sensitive point appears at the small intestine area, usually pathological organic development in the heart can be excluded, and very likely it can be insomnia, palpitation, or other syndrome caused by discordance between the heart and kidney. This method of analysis is commonly used in clinical application.

(2) Analysis based on modern medical science. For example, a patient of duodenal ulcer shows the pain sensitive point at the duodenum point of his auricle. In anatomy, duodenum is controlled by the vegetative nervous system, and pain caused by duodenal ulcer inevitably affects the sympathetic nerve, so that the sympathetic point at the auricle shows pain sensitivity. Pain caused by duodenal ulcer often spreads over the patient's side and back, so the lumbar and sacral vertebra area of the patient's auricle shows pain sensitivity. Finally, based on the theory that an ulcer is caused by disintegration of epithelial tissue, the auricular acupuncture points of dermis and *shen-men* of a patient suffering duodenal ulcer are pain sensitive.

(3) Analysis based on reference acupuncture points of dis-

eases. For those positively diagnosed diseases, carefully examine ear acupuncture points in a large number of cases, clearly record the location of each pain sensitive point, and after statistical computation select several (usually, 3-5) pain sensitive points with higher frequency of appearance. The preliminary assumption is that these acupuncture points which are pain sensitive must be related to certain diseases. Thus, these acupuncture points are called diagnosis reference acupuncture points in overall analysis.

For example, in 52 cases of positively diagnosed nephritis, we proceed to locate pain sensitive auricular points and find their distribution as follows:

TABLE 10-1

Distribution of Auricular Pain Sensitive Points in 52 Cases of Nephritis

Ear Acupuncture Point	Kidney	Bladder	Internal Secretion	Nephritis Point	Ureter	Triple Warmer	Shoulder Joint
frequency	52	51	52	52	25	27	31
Ear Acupuncture Point	Sympathetic	Stomach	Liver	Oesophagus	Lumbago Point	Shenmen	Occiput
frequency	17	31	11	47	43	31	24
Ear Acupuncture Point	Uterus	Suprarenal Gland	Heart	Trachea	Mouth	Eye	Large Intestine
frequency	19	19	21	19	21	11	21

Table 10-1 shows that in 52 cases of nephritis the acupuncture points of kidney, bladder, internal secretion, and nephritis point show pain sensitivity more than 51 times. This suggests that the four pain sensitive points have definite relationship with nephritis. Therefore, these four acupuncture points are diagnosis reference points in diagnosing nephritis.

By carrying out an examination of a large number of ear acupuncture points, we can discover patterns of each type of disease. If this method can be used to compare and contrast an equal number of cases (such as comparison of nephritis and non-nephritis patients), the diagnosis reference acupuncture points so determined will be more valuable. Although we have done some work in this field, we do not have a sufficiently large number of cases. The following table of diagnosis reference acupuncture points for common diseases is prepared for further research.

TABLE 10-2
Diagnosis Reference Acupuncture Points for Common Diseases

No.	Disease	Primary Acu- puncture Points	Secondary Acu- puncture Points	Remarks
1	hepatitis	**hepatitis area, hepatitis point**	internal secre- tion, sympathetic	
		liver yang$_1$, *liver yang*$_2$,		maybe malfunc- tion of liver
2	hepatomegalia	**hepatomegalia area, triple warmer**		often seen at right auricle
3	schistosomiasis	**schistosoma sensitive line**	large intestine	often seen at right auricle
4	inflammation of gall bladder	**gall, outer abdomen**	stomach, liver, shoulder	often seen at right auricle
5	appendicitis	**appendix**	large intestine, triple warmer	often seen at right auricle
6	hypertrophic spinitis	**corresponding area**	kidney	at both auricles
7	nephritis	**kidney, nephritis point**	bladder, internal secretion	same
8	kidney pyelitis	**nephritis point, external genital, urethra, kidney**	bladder, internal secretion	same
9	constipation	**constipation**	large intestine	same
10	hemorrhoid	**constipation, lower section of rectum**	large intestine, triple warmer	same
11	neurasthenia	**dermis,** *shen-men*	heart	same
12	mastitis	**thorax, mammary gland**	internal secretion	often seen on same side
13	asthma	**bronchus**	asthma point, asthma	
14	cirrhosis	**muscle relax point, hepato- megalia area**	stomach, oesophagus	
15	lessening male sexual function	**testicle, uterus**	excitement point	
16	gastritis	**stomach, oesophagus**	cardia, small intestine	

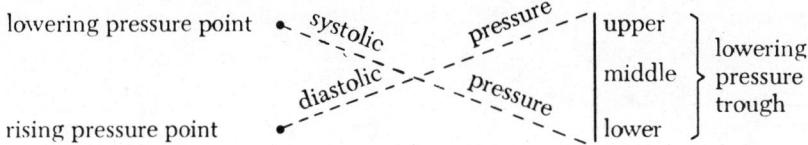

lowering pressure point

rising pressure point

upper ⎫
middle ⎬ lowering pressure trough
lower ⎭

FIGURE 10-2   Blood Pressure Indicator

TABLE 10-3

Diagnosis Reference Acupuncture Points for Blood Pressure

Range of Blood Pressure		Rising Pressure Point	Lowering Pressure Point	Lowering Pressure Trough		
				Upper	Middle	Lower
90/60 mm. mercury column	±5	+	−	+	−	−
130/90 mm. mercury column	±5	+	+	±	−	**+**
140/100 mm. mercury column	±5	±	+	±±	−	±
150/110 mm. mercury column	±5	±±	+	±±	−	±
180/120 mm. mercury column	±5	±±	±±	+	±±	+

Note: + means sound; ± sound plus pricking pain; ++ louder sound;
       ±± louder sound plus pricking pain.

Case Studies

Case 1: Li, male, age 36, formerly engineer of an air force unit.

Patient's complaint: persistent lumbago for several years; more severe in rainy weather and winter time; no obvious effect after repeated treatment by both traditional and modern doctors.

Record of auricular sensitive points examination:

Right auricle: *shen-men,* **uterus, lumbago point, lumbar verte-bra**[1,2], lumbar and sacral vertebra, **kidney,** stomach, shoulder joint, temple, occiput, forehead, testicle, hepatomegalia (lower), knee joint, bronchus, sympathetic, dermis.

Left auricle: hepatomegalia (lower), bronchus, **lumbago point,**

kidney, other points same as on the right auricle.

Analysis based on both pathological history and auricular acupuncture points reaction:

First consideration for lumbago is vertebra: lumbago point, lumbar vertebra$_{1,2}$, and lumbar and sacral vertebra. The three sensitive points suggest pathological location in lumbar vertebra$_{1,2}$, in agreement with patient's complaint.

Also at the kidney point there is a clear pricking pain. According to the theory "kidneys control bone" in traditional Chinese medicine, the disease appears to be not functional. Other cases show that debilitating diseases such as broken bones, osteal tuberculosis, periostitis, and osteoma cause strong reaction at the kidney point. Thus, in the present case, lumbago may be caused by pathological development in bones, and it is located at the lumbar vertebra$_{1,2}$ area. Many diseases of the bones may cause lumbago, such as osteal tuberculosis, sprained joints, and broken bones, but in the case of osteal tuberculosis, the upper and lower tubercle points in the heart area may have a *yang* reaction. Since this case does not have such a reaction, this disease can be excluded. In cases of sprained joints and broken bones, there must have been external injury, but the patient reports no such occurrence. When all these conditions are considered, the possibility for inflammation of lumbar vertebra is good. Its inflamed location is at the lumbar vertebra$_{1,2}$ area.

Secondly, usually when a male patient suffers neurasthenia and obstruction of sexual function, his uterus point is pain sensitive. In this case, both uterus and testicle are sensitive, and uterus feels pricking pain. According to statistical data, if the above two points of a male patient in the age bracket of 30 to 40 show sensitivity, the possibility for obstruction of sexual function (such as impotence and premature spermatorrhea) is good. But this case shows lumbar aching on both sides, while lumbago is unclear.

Thirdly, lumbago may also be related to liver diseases. The appearance of a sensitive point at hepatomegalia area (lower area) suggests hepatomegalia, but by itself it is not conclusive evidence for liver disease (other symptoms are pain at right upper abdomen, loss of appetite, and no taste for greasy food). Then examine the hepatitis point, hepatitis area, liver $yang_1$, and liver $yang_2$, and find these acupuncture points not sensitive. Thus, hepatitis can be excluded. The only possibility is simple mild hepatomegalia (about 1-1.5 cm.), but this is insufficient to cause lumbago.

The question of pain sensitive points at the sympathetic and stomach is solved by examining other acupuncture points of the gastric and digestive system and find them not pain sensitive. Thus, the possibility for diseases of the digestive system are unlikely.

The appearance of sensitive points at the temple, dermis, forehead, and *shen-men* suggests headache, dizzy spells, insomnia, and lack of strength, all belonging to a functional syndrome.

The preliminary diagnosis of the present case is summed up as follows:

(1) Lumbago is caused by hypertrophic vertebritis (lumbar $vertebra_{1,2}$).

(2) Lessening sexual function, rising deficient *yang* accompanied by dizziness, insomnia, and indigestion.

(3) Hepatomegalia by 1-1.5 cm., while liver function is normal.

The above preliminary diagnosis was confirmed at a hospital in Nanking.

Case 2: Hsu, male, age 64, retired cadre.

Patient's complaint: fortnight ago, sudden hemoptysis, tarry stool, accompanied by dizziness and lack of strength; no abdominal pain; no history of stomachache.

Record of auricular sensitive points examination:

Right auricle: uterus, **stomach, cardia, dermis, internal secretion, suprarenal gland, tonsil$_4$-helix$_4$ line,** heart, occiput, mouth, oesophagus.

Analysis based on both pathological history and auricular acupuncture points reaction:

Tarry stool and hemoptysis suggest hemorrhage of the upper digestive system. Pricking pain at both stomach and cardia points further confirms the disease as one of the digestive system. Since the patient has no history of stomachache and the two points of sympathetic and lumbar and sacral vertebra are not sensitive, the possibility for chronic ulcer is unlikely.

The fact that internal secretion, dermis, and suprarenal gland, and the tonsil4-helix4 line feel clear pricking pain suggests a case of malignant tumor[1], and its location is somewhere between the cardia and the stomach area.

Analysis based on both auricular acupuncture points reaction and patient's pathological history:

It is a case of cardiac cancer or gastric cancer.

Later, the patient's alimentary canal was examined by barium meal test in No. 2 Hospital of the Nanking Medical School and confirmed as cardiac cancer in gastric oesophagus.

Case 3: Fan, male, age 34, factory technician.

The patient asked for a health check and wanted to find out about the accuracy of the ear acupuncture points locating device in disease diagnosis.

Record of auricle sensitive points examination:

Shen-men, dermis, lowering pressure point +, rising pressure point +, upper section of lowering pressure trough +, lower section of lowering pressure trough +, bronchus, throat, sympathetic, **stomach,** occiput, shoulder joint, toothache point, tooth extraction anaesthesia point, triple warmer, constipation, large intestine, lumbago point, oesophagus.

Analysis based on the sensitive points is summed up as follows:

The sensitive points of dermis and *shen-men* are caused by pain. That acupuncture points of the sympathetic, triple warmer, stomach, and oesophagus are sensitive and the stomach point feels pricking pain suggests pain related to the stomach area, and is thus considered a good possibility of gastritis.

---

[1] In 82 cases of confirmed diagnosis of a variety of tumors, 80 patients' acupuncture points of suprarenal gland, internal secretion, and dermis, and the narrow belt between tonsil4 and helix4 were sensitive. The instrument showed that these sensitive points of most patients transmit sound and feel pricking pain, and those of a few others transmit less audible sound but feel pricking pain. Besides, in cases of tumor in abdominal cavity and cancer of oesophagus, no sensitive reaction is detected in the above-mentioned areas. In recent years, we had discussions with other units, and they also discovered that the above patterns fit some patients with tumor. The above three points and one line can be used for reference in diagnosis. In clinical application, however, we also discovered that some patients showed clear reaction in the above mentioned areas, but other tests proved them not tumor patients. Therefore, in auricular diagnosis of this disease, a patient's history, repeated tests, and careful analysis are required, while any hasty conclusion should be avoided.

The fact that lowering pressure point +, rising pressure point +, upper section of lowering pressure trough +, and lower section of lowering pressure trough + suggests, according to Table 10-2, that the patient's blood pressure is about 130/90 mm. mercury column.

The toothache point and tooth extraction anaesthesia point sensitivity may be caused by gingivitis, pulpitis, or a decayed or broken tooth.

That constiptation and large intestine, temple and forehead area, and lumbago points are sensitive suggests that the patient has obstipation, dizziness, and lumbar ache.

The appearance of sensitive points at the bronchus and throat, considered along with the sensitive points of *shen-men* and sympathetic, suggests pharyngitis and bronchitis. But the two points of the bronchus and throat feel no clear pricking pain and show no visible skin change, so that they are advanced diseases of chronic nature.

Preliminary summary:

(1) blood pressure 130/90 mm. mercury column; (2) chronic gastritis; (3) chronic pharyngitis and chronic bronchitis; (4) toothache or broken tooth; (5) obstipation, dizziness, and lumbar ache.

Recounting pathological history:

(1) The patient suffered gastritis with excessive gastric acid and poor digestion in 1958. No unusual discovery was made after several barium meal tests. He has a long history of trachitis and coughs often.

(2) Before undergoing an auricular acupuncture points examination, he went to a clinic with his blood pressure measured at 128/90 mm. mercury column.

(3) Other symptoms confirm the result of auricular acupuncture points diagnosis.

Case 4: Chu, female, age 41, soldier.

This patient traveled all the way from Anhwei to Nanking for an ear acupuncture points examination and diagnosis.

Record of auricular sensitive points examination:

Right auricle: *shen-men*, **uterus**, lowering pressure point —,

hepatitis point, hepatitis area, kidney, sympathetic, **hepatomegalia area,** lung area, internal secretion, **external genital,** liver $yang_1$, rising pressure point +, upper section of lowering pressure trough +, oesophagus, stomach, lumbago point, triple warmer, shoulder joint, pelvis cavum, dermis.

Analysis of the sensitive points:

When too many sensitive points are found in auricular examination, these points should be classified and analyzed step by step.

In this case, five points—**hepatitis area,** liver $yang_1$, **hepatitis point,** internal secretion, and sympathetic—are sensitive, which suggest hepatitis.[2]

Since liver $yang_2$ and ascites point show no reaction, it is chronic hepatitis, and the liver function is normal.

The appearance of sensitive points at the hepatomegalia area and the center point of the lower zone of the right auricle suggests hepatomegalia (beneath ribs) by about 2.5 cm.

The sensitive points of the stomach and oesophagus are caused by discord between the liver and stomach as a result of chronic hepatitis, stomach disorder, and abdominal distention.

The sensitive points of *shen-men*, dermis, and triple warmer suggest pain in the liver area.

The three sensitive points of **uterus, external genital,** and pelvis cavum often appear in gynecological diseases and possibly suggest cervicitis.

Although the bronchus part of the lung area is sensitive, the patient feels no pricking pain. It may be caused by chronic pathological development of the bronchus.

Dizziness caused by hepatitis is often shown at the sensitive points of the forehead and temple, but very few patients have a sensitive lumbago point. After inquiry, it is learned that the patient suffered a strained lumbar and still felt lumbago recently.

After the auricular examination, the patient was asked about her pathological history, health check, and other special check-ups.

Patient's complaint: 12 years of hepatitis; malignant pneu-

---

[2] In 115 confirmed cases of hepatitis, more than 80% show that the five points are sensitive.

monia in 1969 and coughing occasionally at present; excessive leukorrhea.

Health check record: blood pressure 96/58 mm. mercury column; hepatomegalia (beneath ribs) by 2-3 cm, slight pain when touched.

Liver function: normal.

Ultra-sonic vibrations: in liver area, 2.5 cm. beneath ribs.

Case 5: Mrs. Lu (nee Li), age 69, female, native of Ningpo.

Patient's complaint: abdominal pain, sometimes acute, resistance to food, confined to bed for a week.

Preliminary examination in one hospital suggests: (1) acute gastritis? (2) stomach cancer? Later, she is transferred to our unit for auricular sensitive points examination.

Record of auricular sensitive points examination:

Gall, liver, stomach, abdomen, occiput, internal secretion, sympathetic, *shen-men,* dermis, outer abdomen.

Analysis based on patient's pathological history, the record of preliminary examination in the other hospital, and the record of auricular sensitive points examination:

Patient suffering gastritis usually shows sensitive points at oesophagus, cardia, stomach, and duodenum around crus of helix. In this case the patient suffers abdominal pain and refuses food that suggests pathological development of the digestive system related to the stomach area. Auricular examination shows that the gall area is sensitive and feels sharper pricking pain than the stomach area. According to the statistical data about gall bladder inflammation,[3] the patient's abdominal pain may be caused by gall bladder inflammation rather than gastritis.

The possibility of stomach cancer, viewed from the distribution of the auricular sensitive points, is rather unlikely.

On July 3, 1971, the patient was examined, tested, and her gall bladder X-rayed in Shanghai Juichin Hospital and diagnosed a case of sudden onset of chronic gall bladder inflammation.

In the past several years, we have applied the ear acupuncture

---

3 In 24 confirmed cases of gall bladder inflammation, 21 showed that the gall area, liver, and outer abdomen are sensitive, and the gall area feels pricking pain.

points locating device to clinical use with success, but many problems remain for us to explore further. For instance, people hold different views of the sensitive point, and more advanced research and analysis are required to understand its significance. Moreover, additional study is needed for improvement of the ear acupuncture points locating device. Since the reason for the appearance of the sensitive point is yet to be further studied, the design of the instrument cannot be simply based on the one factor of variable electric resistance condition of skin. After a certain period of application, we realized that change of ear acupuncture point sensitivity is shown not only in variable electric resistance but also in variable electric potential. We discovered that the electric potential of the sensitive point is larger than that of the normal ear acupuncture point. This has great impact on the auricular sensitive points locating device designed on the basis of alternating electric current signals because the volume of electric potential is closely related to frequency of sound signals. At present, not sufficient data is available to support this work, but it will be a worthy research topic for those engaged in the design of medical instruments.

CHAPTER 11

The Use of the Dialectical Method in Selecting Acupuncture Points in Clinical Application

In clinical application of ear acupuncture, great emphasis is placed on the dialectical method in selecting acupuncture points. Whether the acupuncturist can correctly understand the dialectical method in selecting acupuncture points in clinical treatment will greatly affect restoration to health. If he can, the treatment will be effective. Otherwise, the treatment will be less effective or not effective at all.

We encountered a patient who suffered stomach ulcer for four years and his stomach suffered hunger pain. For a long time, he could not eat well. If he ate too much, his stomach felt uncomfortable. If he ate too little, his stomach felt pain, often accompained by gastric distention. His complexion was sallow, and his four limbs suffered aching pain and were weak. Surgery was recommended at several hospitals. But the patient was unwilling to undergo an operation and wanted ear acupuncture treatment. Stomach ulcer is a common disease of the alimentary canal, and we decided to treat the disease according to the main syndrome. The acupuncture points we chose were sympathetic, *shen-men*, stomach, and dermis. After needling three times, the patient felt less pain, his appetite was improved, and his abdominal distention also relieved. Since then, his condition was severe sometimes and sometimes mild, good sometimes and sometimes bad. The patient underwent three series of treatment, or a total of 32 insertions. Although his condition was relieved and checked, it was not completely cured. The patient asked us to continue the treatment. We also felt that since his condition was improved, his complexion turned from sallow to healthy red, and his limbs gained strength, there was an element of cure in the treatment.

We then proceeded, on the basis of the patient's syndrome, to consult references about the disease in both traditional Chinese medical knowledge and modern medical science and to analyze, together with the patient, the daily record of the past 32 insertions. We concluded that the combination of acupuncture points we chose aimed directly at the disease and lacked the dialectical method of treatment in traditional Chinese medicine. We then decided to select acupuncture points of sympathetic, shenmen, stomach, spleen, and lung, according to the principle of "strengthen spleen to assist stomach; help good to correct evil" in traditional Chinese medicine. Here the main purpose was "strengthen spleen and help good" with the resulting effect of "assist stomach and correct evil." The earlier approach, from the selection of acupuncture points to the treatment itself, was aimed directly at curing the disease. Therefore, the patient only had some relief of his condition. Chairman Mao has taught us: "The quality of a thing is mainly determined by the principal aspect of the contradiction that has won the dominant position. When the principal aspect of the contradiction which has won the dominant position undergoes a change, the quality of a thing changes accordingly." In selecting the new combination of acupuncture points, we grasped the principal aspect of the contradiction to focus on strengthening the spleen. We increased the stimulation of the spleen point by inserting several needles while lessening the stimulation at the stomach point. After needling three times, the patient's stomachache and abdominal distention disappeared and his appetite was clearly improved. After needling 14 times, the stomach was X-rayed. Originally, the almond-sized ulcer at the curved section of the stomach completely disappeared, and the patient was totally cured.

Why did the alteration of several acupuncture points effect a cure? We believe that it was because on the basis of the dialectic treatment method in traditional Chinese medicine we grasped the principal aspect of the contradiction, that is, strengthening the spleen, to take a qualitative leap from the original method of treatment. In the process of treating this patient of stomach ulcer, we deepened our understanding of the dialectical method in selecting acupuncture points and came to realize the dialectical relationship between the selection of different acupuncture points and different ear acupuncture approaches for a variety of diseases.

In another case, a patient had chronic bacterial dysentery for more than ten years. He suffered abdominal pain, distention, irregular bowel movements, lack of appetite, and weakened conditions. He was hospitalized several times and for more than two years at one time. While in the hospital despite the use of all kinds of medicines and a number of treatments, he was never totally cured. A routine examination of stool showed red (blood) cell + +, pus cell + +———+ + +, and positive stool culture. We lacked experience in treating this kind of chronic disease, but with the active cooperation of the patient we chose to deal with abdominal distention and abdominal pain. The combination of acupuncture points we chose was: sympathetic, *shen-men*, large intestine, small intestine, and abdomen. After a series of treatment, only the abdominal pain was somehow relieved, but the treatment was not effective. We analyzed the combination of acupuncture points in the treatment along with the patient's pathological history and felt that after years of protracted chronic dysentery, the mucous membrane of the large intestine infected with chronic ulcer and edema was difficult to cure. In addition, because of the prolonged use of medicine, resistance to drugs was built up. This kind of chronic disease could not be cured within a short period. According to traditional Chinese medicine, a long period of loose bowel movements enfeebles intestines, and for treatment the enfeebled should be strengthened and the deteriorated consolidated. According to diagnosis and treatment of similar cases both in traditional Chinese medicine and modern medical science, we decided to omit *shen-men* and the abdomen from the earlier combination of acupuncture points (according to clinical experience, needling the *shen-men* point may increase abdominal distention), and added two new points—the lung and heart (because the viscera theory of traditional Chinese medicine tells us that the lung and large intestine are intimately related, and so are the heart and small intestine). Clinical application had shown that needling the lung point was more effective in treating ulcer. This way after needling twice, the patient's abdominal pain and distention disappeared, and his appetite improved. After needling 10 times, the patient was free of all diseases and his stool culture turned negative. We gave him another series of treatment for building body resistance. After that, this patient of a decade of protracted, chronic dysentery, was completely cured.

Dialectical selection of acupuncture points is a method based on the viscera dialectical method in traditional Chinese medicine to comprehensively understand the cause, location, characteristics, and tendency of a disease in order to grasp the essence of the disease and to determine the proper combination of acupuncture points. In deciding on the combination of acupuncture points, we must correctly handle the dialectical relationship between primary and secondary acupuncture points.

The origin and development of disease is the result of the struggle and transformation of contradictions in the organic body. The human body is a unified whole, and the brain, nerves, internal organs, and limbs are interrelated and interrestrained. The development of any disease is by no means an isolated incident, but is restrained and affected by a variety of factors. Among these factors only one contradiction is of primary and decisive importance while the rest are secondary. "The dialectical world outlook teaches man chiefly how to observe and analyze skillfully the movement of opposites in various things and, on the basis of such analysis, to find out the methods of solving the contradictions." The dialectical selection of points in ear acupuncture is to identify the relationship between the disease and the organic body, to identify the primary and secondary contradictions. When the primary and the secondary are handled properly, we can treat disease by inserting needles into correct acupuncture points. We can then cause the transformation of contradictions, maintain control in the process of treatment, cure disease, and restore the patient's health.

According to our preliminary understanding, there are three guiding principles in selecting ear acupuncture points.

(1) Selection of acupuncture points according to corresponding areas: The pathological development of the intestines and limbs is shown in pain sensitive points on the auricle. For instance, in treating stomachache, insert the needle into the sensitive stomach point at the diminishing area of crus of helix. For fractured collarbone, insert the needle into the collarbone point in scaphoid fossa. This is the method of needling the corresponding area. This method is effective in treating some acute diseases.

(2) Selection of acupuncture points according to the dialectical method in traditional Chinese medicine: By applying the viscera theory of traditional Chinese medicine in clinical use, we may not make the mistake of "treating the head because of headache and treating the foot because of foot pain." The viscera theory of traditional Chinese medicine, such as the intimate relationship between the heart and small intestine, lung and large intestine, kidney and bladder, stomach and spleen, liver and gall, sounds inscrutable but proves effective in clinical application. The efficacy of the theory in disease treatment is a fact. For instance, a patient suffering diseases of the cardiovascular system shows a reaction at the small intestine point, and it will be more effective in treating cardiovascular disease by also needling the secondary acupuncture point of the small intestine. For treating indigestion and functional disorder of the intestines, the use of the secondary acupuncture point of the heart will also increase efficacy. Again, according to the traditional Chinese medical theory "the orifice of the kidney is the ear," we use the kidney point in treating diseases such as tinnitis aurium and otitis media with outstanding curing effects.

(3) Selection of acupuncture points according to the function of commonly used points and clinical experience: The selection of commonly used acupuncture points and acupuncture points

based on clinical experience depends on a large number of case studies. Otherwise, difficulties will be encountered in the process of treatment.

Furthermore, in clinical application, it is better to select fewer but more effective acupuncture points. Generally speaking, use the auricular acupuncture points of the suffering side; in a few cases use those of the opposite side. When necessary, for improving efficacy, use acupuncture points of both sides.

CHAPTER 12

How to Maintain Control in the Course of Treatment

Chairman Mao has taught us: "The process of change in the objective world will never end, nor will man's knowledge of truth through practice." In using ear acupuncture treatment to serve workers, peasants, and soldiers, we took as a guiding principle Chairman Mao's brilliant idea "practice, knowledge, more practice, more knowledge." We gave priority to practice, maintained initiative, and stressed change—changing "incurable" to "curable"—to maintain control in treatment of rare and difficult diseases.

Control of "Recurrence" and Maintaining Initiative

There is a certain view: ear acupuncture treatment is effective in treating acute diseases but incapable of real cure of chronic diseases which show tendency of recurrence. Does fact really bear out this assertion? There was a patient who suffered chronic enteritis, felt abdominal pain and distention daily, and discharged whatever he ate. After the failure of all kinds of treatment, he came to us for ear acupuncture treatment. At the beginning we selected a combination of four points—sympathetic, *shen-men*, large intestine, and small intestine.. The goal was to kill pain and halt diarrhea. After the first insertion, the patient no longer felt abdominal pain.

After the second insertion, his abdominal distention disappeared, his bowel movements turned normal, and his appetite was improved. After the sixth insertion, he ate two pieces of watermelon and an apple without any negative effect. At that time, the patient was very happy, for he felt that his disease was gone. We also believed that it was about cured and ended the treatment after a total of eight insertions. Unexpectedly, two weeks later the patient again suffered abdominal distention and diarrhea. On the basis of the symptoms, our diagnosis was recurrence at the initial stage, for the patient suffered mild abdominal distention, fewer loose bowel movements, and no abdominal pain. Using the same acupuncture points, we gave him another treatment, and the above symptoms quickly disappeared. But one month after stopping acupuncture treatment, because of careless eating and drinking, the patient once more suffered diarrhea and came for continual treatment. We studied the symptoms of the two recurrences and found them milder each time. But his condition after two treatments showed that his intestinal function had not fundamentally recovered. Therefore, we gave him two more insertions to consolidate his intestinal function. After that, all symptoms disappeared, and for more than a year the patient's condition remained good.

Chairman Mao once said: "We must encourage thinking, learn the method of analysis and cultivate the habit of analysis." In line with this teaching, we further analyzed the patterns of two recurrences together with the patient. We found the symptoms of the first recurrence were different from those before the treatment, such as no abdominal pain, mild abdominal distention, and fewer loose bowel movements. Comparing the two recurrences, the conditions of the second recurrence also differed from those of the first, that is, there was no abdominal pain and distention and only mild diarrhea. This means that "recurrence" was a case of improvement, a normal phenomenon in the process of treatment. That shows there is a process of development from quantitative change to qualitative change. "In judging the trueness of one's knowledge or theory, one cannot depend upon one's subjective feelings about it, but upon its objective result in social practice." Does our understanding of "recurrence" correspond to objective reality? Using past cases, we made a statistical study of a certain period and discovered that in the process of treatment, cases of "recurrence" amounted to more than one-third or nearly one-half. This was so especially in diseases of the nervous system, diseases of the urinary and reproductory system, and skin diseases. In some cases the "recurrence" period was short, while in others long. Based on this finding, we made a classification of the "recurrence" phenomena of a large variety of diseases, and carefully studied each category in order to understand the development of "recurrence."

For example, there was a patient of sebaceous dermatitis. After several periods of insertion, he stopped losing hair. A short while after stopping treatment, he again started losing hair. When the treatment was resumed, he stopped losing hair again. When it was stopped, the disease recurred. After this pattern of repetition, our confidence was shaken. But the patient insisted that he was cured after the third series of insertions. This process of "recurrence" inspired us to give the phenomenon careful consideration. In the past, in the process of treating some diseases if no obvious effect was observed or "recurrence" appeared, we thought that ear acupuncture treatment was "unsuitable." Either the physician gave up treatment or the patient did not want to continue. Actually, "suitable" or "unsuitable," "curable" or "incurable" is not absolute, not unchangeable. It is mainly because we have not fully understood the intrinsic laws of the disease. The reason is perhaps an unsuitable combination of primary and secondary acupuncture points, or insufficient length of treatment, or "stages of development" in the disease itself, or other factors in the method of treatment. Once we master these intrinsic laws and improve our method of treatment, according to the characteristics of the disease, then "unsuitable" will turn into "suitable." If we fail to recognize this, then as soon as we encounter "recurrence" or other difficulties, we may hastily conclude that ear acupuncture does not fit a particular disease; thus blinded by our own prejudice, we make mistakes in our treatment.

Chairman Mao once said: "What Marxist philosophy regards as the most important problem does not lie in understanding the laws of the objective world and thereby becoming capable of explaining it, but in actively changing the world by applying the knowledge of its objective laws." We reason: since "recurrence" appears in the course of treatment, can it be solved in the course of treatment? Can we maintain the initiative? Can we change severe "recurrence" to mild "recurrence," change many "recurrences" to few "recurrences," change "recurrence" to "no recurrence?"

We gained inspiration after treating a patient of high blood pressure. In the past, when we treated patients of high blood pressure with ear acupuncture, our goal was to lower the blood pressure and to relieve the condition. Therefore, we usually stopped treatment after insertion several times. But this patient of high blood pressure refused to stop treatment after two or three insertions. Instead, he asked us to give him a complete series of treatment. After two months, he happily informed us that his high blood pressure never recurred. The cure was completely attained by ear acupuncture treatment. Why? Analysis based on treatment data shows that the cure results from leaving the needle in place longer and from inserting it many times. The patient also reported that he underwent ear acupuncture treatment in the past, but not as long as this time. In the past, needling off and on only had a relieving effect for a day or two, but had no complete curing effect. He failed to insist on prolonged treatment. The case shows that the fewer times the insertions, the shorter the duration of efficacy. On the other hand, the more times the insertions, the longer the duration of cure. But would continual treatment with longer treatment period and more times of insertion increase the efficacy of treatment? What would happen if this hypothesis is applied to some diseases susceptible to recurrence? Would this method reduce the number of "recurrences" or even eliminate "recurrence" once and for all?

We tested this hypothesis first in some diseases of the nervous system which are susceptible to "recurrence." One method was to change a short to a longer treatment period, that is, to change the original treatment period of ten times to a longer treatment period of 15 or 20 times. Another method was to shorten the interval between treatments from 5-7 days to 3-5 days. A third method was to eliminate the interval between treatments. Usually, when one treatment period was completed the patient rested for several days, primarily for recovery from "acupuncture point fatigue." Now it was changed to needle insertion every other day. This way "acupuncture point fatigue" was taken care of and the possibility of recurrence during the interval between treatments was avoided. As a result, most diseases susceptible to "recurrence" had fewer "recurrences," or even no "recurrence" at all. We further applied the hypothesis and methods to other diseases, and their "recurrences" were also greatly reduced. Thus, we reached a new understanding and opened a new path in shortening the overall duration of treatment and to make cures more effective.

Reliance on Practice; Courage to Face Challenge

In our clinical practice, we often encountered some rare and difficult diseases. Our attitude toward such diseases is neither shun responsibility nor worry about results. We persist in practice to grope for new methods of treatment. We believe that no matter how difficult a disease is, there must be some way to cure it, and the only way to find the proper method is through practice. Wisdom originates in practice, and the only way to cure a disease is to accept the challenge.

We encountered a patient of a "unique" disease—pulselessness —whose collateral arteries on both sides lost pulse and whose two upper limbs lost blood pressure. He was in this condition for six years and had severe superior paraplegia in the last three years. He was confined to bed year round, unable to take meals, put on clothes, and use the toilet by himself. He sought treatment everywhere, visited many famous doctors, took a variety of medicines, and received many injections to no avail. Finally, he asked us to treat him with ear acupuncture. Pulselessness is a kind of so-called protracted, incurable organic disease. Can ear acupuncture cure this kind of disease? We still maintained the attitude of shunning no responsibility and of not worrying about results.

After detailed inquiry of the patient's pathological history, careful study of his conditions, thorough research of references about the disease in both traditional Chinese medicine and modern medical science, and repeated group discussions, we decided to make the best use of the function of ear acupuncture in regulating body organism and to start with stimulating vasodilatation. We adopted a treating method of "heart strengthening combined acupuncture points," focusing on the acupuncture points of the heart, sympathetic, suprarenal gland, collar bone, dermis, and kidney. The initial result suggested that this method completely fitted the patient's conditions. After needling several times, the patient felt relief all over his body, and his condition improved. Since then, he was no longer taken to the hospital on an ambulance, but walked in with the support of his daughter. After several more acupuncture treatments, he came by himself with the support of a crutch. After one series of treatment, this pulseless patient pronounced "dead" by a few medical authorities regained normal pulse after six years of no pulse. Thereafter, he received more than a month of supporting treatment, and his semi-paralyzed body was totally recovered. Very soon, he returned to work. This case provides us with invaluable experience in treating pulselessness.

Chairman Mao teaches us: "The active function of knowledge not only manifests itself in the active leap from perceptual knowledge to rational knowledge, but also—and this is the more important—in the leap from rational knowledge to revolutionary practice." Therefore, we carefully summarized the successful experience in treating the first case of pulselessness. In three years, we applied the experience to more than 40 cases of pulselessness and established that the method of "heart strengthening combined acupuncture points" fits pulselessness and obtains good curing results. But "contradiction exists in the process of development of all things," and there are numerous variations in objective realities. One case of pulselessness differs from another, for each is developed from its particularity and manifests in a number of different symptoms. We must realize the numerous variations and grasp each particularity. Each patient should be treated differently and each disease dealt with differently. We should not regard the use of a certain combination of acupuncture points for treating a certain disease as an absolute "law."

We treated the following two cases. One was a young worker who had a mild case of pulselessness for a short period. With the experience of treating the above-mentioned case, we thought it should be enough to give him six periods of treatment. Yet after 11 treatments, no effect was shown. Why? The problem lay in the use of types of needles for primary and secondary acupuncture points as well as in the method of inserting needles. The needles we used were all thin ones which produced insufficient stimulation for a young, stout worker. We then changed to thick needles for primary acupuncture points and used a different method of insertion to produce stronger stimulation. After needling twice, his artery regained pulse.

Another was an office worker over forty years old who suffered pulselessness accompanied by irregular heart rhythm, palpitation, and short breath. As soon as several needles were inserted, the patient's collateral artery of the affected area showed pulse, and blood pressure was also detected. Unexpectedly, however, after half an hour, the patient suffered a dizzy spell and palpitation, and his cervical artery of the affected area produced a full pulse up to more than 150 beats per minute. We quickly pulled out the needles, and after two minutes the patient returned to normal. Therefore, we proceeded to analyze one by one the combination of acupuncture points. We realized that the suprarenal gland point in the combination of "heart strengthening acupuncture points" was not suitable for a weak and older patient of pulselessness with a heart ailment. This acupuncture point increases blood pressure and accelerates pulsation. After we omitted this acupuncture point, the above reactions did not reappear.

The two cases further deepen our understanding of pulselessness. We continually summarize clinical experiences and actively apply them to future clinical treatment so that we learn to use different methods for treating similar diseases with different symptoms. In the development of using "heart strengthening combined acupuncture points" in 20 cases of pulselessness, at first we only used the combination of acupuncture points of the heart, sympathetic, suprarenal gland, and corresponding area and found it effective within an anticipated period of treatment in most cases. Our understanding of these acupuncture points is as follows:

Heart: In traditional Chinese medicine, there is the theory that the flower of the heart is the face, and the heart supplies blood vessels (with blood). We see a direct relationship between the heart and blood vessels, the heart having the function of supplying blood vessels with blood, promoting blood circulation, and regulating the elastic function of vessel wall. We have observed that in clinical treatment, when the heart point is inserted with a needle, the patient's pulse shows a stronger beat. Therefore, the heart point plays a very important role in an "overall heart strengthening" function.

Sympathetic: It has the function of regulating vegetative nerve and distending blood vessels.

Suprarenal Gland: It has the function of increasing the volume of blood circulation, raising blood pressure, and speeding up heart rhythm. It also strengthens the resistance capacity of the body and counteracts rheumatism.

Corresponding Area: It is an indispensable acupuncture point in improving local function. It has an internal relationship with the above acupuncture points. Our experience shows that after inserting a needle into the corresponding area, the pulse is quickly strengthened.

The functions of the above four acupuncture points are identified through our treatment of cases of pulselessness. Aside from the function of each individual point, there is the function of interrelationship and interactivation. When the body is viewed as an organic entity, their functions are far more than those stated above. But in application sometimes they do not work as expected. Therefore, we have to make some revision in treating different cases. For instance, a patient with pulselessness and a cardiac ailment, needling his suprarenal gland point will result in an accelerated heart rhythm and a particularly full pulse beat of the blood vessel in the affected part, that the patient cannot endure. For such patients, instead of using the suprarenal gland, we use the kidney and small intestine. The small intestine is intimately related to the heart, and it has the function of compensating the heart. According to traditional Chinese medicine, the heart and kidney have a functional relationship, and the kidney has a strengthening function. Therefore, needling the kidney point counteracts the pulseless patient's dizzy spell, hazy vision, and limb asthenia and invigorates all active elements of his body to strengthen it. For some patients with a prolonged ailment who have undergone different treatments, or even have their sympathetic ganglion excised, or have used hormones for a long time, we also add three acupuncture points of the liver, spleen, and internal secretion in order to balance air and blood circulation. Besides, the liver and spleen have an intimate relationship with sinew and muscle. Thus, inserting needles into these three acupuncture points improves the patient's numbness and asthenia of his affected limbs. In addition to the above points, the brain point and dermis which regulate secretory function of the nervous system are also to be used as secondary points.

On the basis of experience in treating pulselessness, we learn to treat obstructive vasculitis with good results.

Overcoming "Stalemate" During Treatment

In the process of ear acupuncture treatment, we also came across the phenomenon that most patients quickly showed different degrees of cure, but as we proceeded, there was no further improvement after a certain stage. This phenomenon of "stalemate" in the process of treatment often hampered the cure of rare and difficult diseases.

Chairman Mao once said: "All contradictions are objective existence, and our job is to do our best to correctly identify them and to solve them." We used Chairman Mao's philosophical thought to carry out thorough analysis of the "stalemate" phenomenon in rare and difficult diseases. Through analysis, we reason: the human body is a system of unity of opposites, and the opposite sides maintain relative balance to sustain body health. When one side or any part of one side loses balance because of a certain factor, the body becomes ill. Everything undergoes change. Disease itself too undergoes change. Treatment simply means to create conditions to cause a change for the better. Therefore, even if progress is slow in rare and difficult cases, the phenomenon itself contains an element of change toward balance. The temporary phenomenon of "stalemate" suggests that the conditions we provide for change are insufficient. We should never think that the limited degree of cure is "final," nor should we be satisfied with the attained result. Our responsibility is to make the best use of the regulatory capacity of ear acupuncture, to use every method to create conditions, to invigorate all positive elements in the body, to speed up its change for the better, and finally to attain the goal of a complete cure.

There was an intellectual who suffered a severe case of neurasthenia. For more than twenty years, he had frequent dizzy spells, aching and weak limbs, poor appetite. severe amnesia, and a lack of balance over excitement and restraint. Every night he had to take several kinds of tranquilizers and sleeping pills to the extent of nearly poisoning himself in order to sleep for two or three hours. Because of prolonged use of sleeping pills, he suffered chronic toxic hepatitis, his health worsened, and his work was affected. He went to the countryside to undergo a period of physical labor because he thought a change of environment would do him good. But his conditions were not improved. The patient looked to ear acupuncture with great hope. According to our experience in treating neurasthenia, we had confidence in treating this case and expected to see good results after several treatments. In the early stage of treatment, the patient showed continual improvement; his dizzy spell was gone, he felt relief all over, and his appetite improved. After the seventh treatment, the patient could sleep for more than three hours without the help of sleeping pills. But thereafter the phenomenon of "stalemate" appeared. There was no new progress after the 10th needling, the 15th needling, the 20th needling, and the 30th needling, or a total of three series of treatments. In the meantime, we tried three combinations of acupuncture points, but the patient's sleeping time never lasted for more than four hours, and sometimes only for two hours. After two months of treatment, our conclusion was that his condition changed for the better and was under control. But the main contradiction was not solved, and there was no qualitative change. How to induce qualitative change, or obvious progress? In order to conquer this insurmountable obstacle, to overcome the "stalemate," we started with an analysis of the different symptoms of the patient, gave consideration to pathological factors of this common disease of neurasthenia, and studied each individual acupuncture point. Acupuncture points such as *shen-men*, occiput, dermis, and the heart are usually effective in regulating excitement or restraint of cerebral cortex, but why had there been no qualitative leap? On the basis of Chairman Mao's discussion of transformation of contradictions, "a change determined by the extent of the increase or decrease in the strength with which each of the two aspects struggles against the other in the development of a thing," we studied some cases where high fever (continued for several days) was cured by the method of blood-letting at helix and ear apex. If this method could reduce prolonged fever, could the same method be used to create conditions for tranquilizing and containing neurasthenia? We then added one acupuncture point to the original combination of acupuncture points, that is, letting a few drops of blood at ear apex. After this treatment, the patient slept for five hours. After three continual treatments, the patient was able not only to take a noon nap but also to sleep for more than six hours at night. We contacted the patient one year later and learned that his weight was increased from 50 kg. to more than 60 kg., his memory improved, and his sleep remained at more than six or seven hours each night.

There was another patient who suffered sequela of meningitis and whose lower limbs suffered stiff paralysis for more than six years. After several treatments, the effect was obvious. The paralyzed patient could walk with support along a wall, but there was not much progress in continual treatment. Chairman Mao teaches us: "Contradiction and struggle are universal, absolute, but the methods for solving contradictions, that is, the forms of struggle, differ according to the differences in the nature of the contradictions." Following his teaching, we analyzed the conditions of the patient and reasoned that the patient's disease had a long history and was severe. If we used the general combination of acupuncture points for treating sequela of meningitis, there would not be much progress. This was because the conditions we created were insufficient for invigorating internal positive elements to cause a change for the better. We reasoned that his crural paralysis was mainly caused by an injured motor center which then lost its normal ability in commanding limbs. Our earlier method of treatment was not enough for an injured motor center to recover its normal commanding ability. Therefore, we decided on a new combination of acupuncture points with dermis, brain stem, occiput, kidney, and liver as primary points. The purpose of needling these points was to strengthen the brain. After several treatments, the anticipated result was attained. The patient could not only stand up but also walked several steps. After a few more treatments, the patient basically recovered.

CHAPTER 13

Case Studies

Anaylsis of Acupuncture Points Which Cured Duodenal Ulcer

Chang, male, age 45, mining work cadre from Anhwei.

The patient suffered duodenal ulcer for more than twenty years. He had undergone a barium meal test, and an almond-size ulcer was detected by X-ray. After each meal, his stomach ached and was full of gastric acid. The pain became unbearable at midnight. If he ate a little more or ate food not easily digestible, his stomachache worsened and spread to his back. Because of prolonged under-nourishment, insomnia, and tarry stool in recent years, he was extremely thin. For more than twenty years, the patient had taken all kinds of medicine and received injections to no avail. In the spring of 1970 his condition worsened, his stomach ached continually, and his alimentary canal bled. At this point, the patient came for ear acupuncture treatment.

Selection of acupuncture points: sympathetic, *shen-men,* duodenum, stomach, lung, and dermis.

Preliminary analysis: Ulcerous pain is usually caused by local irritation which leads to spasms of the stomach and duodenum and inadequate blood circulation in the affected area. According to traditional Chinese medicine, pain is considered the result of insufficient circulation of air and blood. Therefore, the above combination of acupuncture points is selected, first, to kill pain and, then, to improve local condition of nourishment and to recover the function of the ailing organ. The acupuncture points of the sympathetic, *shen-men,* and dermis are selected to regulate the function of the vegetative nerve and cerebral cortex for tranquilizing and pain killing. The acupuncture points of the duodenum and stomach are selected to build resistance of the corresponding organs, to improve their functions, in order to attain new balance. Finally, the acupuncture point of the lung is selected for treating ulcer of mucous membrane.

After seven times of needling the above acupuncture points, the patient felt his gastric acid was clearly reduced and his stomachache disappeared. Thereafter, he underwent four series of treatments and felt all syndrome disappeared. An X-ray examination showed that the ulcerous shade at the duodenum disappeared. The patient said: "For more than twenty years I never felt so good."

Analysis of Acupuncture Points Which Cured Acute Infectious Hepatitis

Chu, male, age 36, worker.

The patient had fever continually for six or seven days. He had no appetite, resented greasy food, lacked strength, and had a yellow complexion. Confirmed diagnosis at one hospital: infectious hepatitis, malfunction of the liver, and S.G.P.T. 300 units. After several treatments, the patient felt his fever gone and his appetite clearly improved. After 10 treatments, the S.G.P.T. was reduced to 68 units, and the jaundice index also reduced from 30 to 14 units. After the second series of treatment, the patient felt relieved and his appetite became normal. A test confirmed his liver function as normal. In the course of treatment, the patient took small amount of vitamins but no other medicine.

Selection of Acupuncture Points: liver, spleen, gall, internal secretion, sympathetic, and liver $yang_{1,2}$.

Preliminary Analysis: The acupuncture point of the liver is selected to control symptoms caused by infectious hepatitis and to assist the recovery of the liver cells. Because the liver and gall are intimately related and have a mutually implementing function, the acupuncture point of gall is therefore selected to lower the jaundice index in jaundice-hepatitis. The acupuncture point of internal secretion is selected to assist the organic function of excretion and absorption and to improve its vicarious function. It is thus considered effective in improving the secretion, excretion, vicarious, and antidotal functions of liver cells.

This combination of acupuncture points is also effective in treating other kinds of hepatitis.

Combination of Acupuncture Points
for Curing Neurasthenia

Hsing, age 48, office cadre.

The patient had neurasthenia for more than twenty years. He could not sleep all night for a long time, occasionally slept for 3-4 hours, and had dizzy spells and headache during the day. For more than twenty years, he could not quit using sleeping pills, his memory was deteriorating, and his work seriously affected. He started undergoing ear acupuncture treatment since November of 1970.

Selection of Acupuncture Points: heart, kidney, dermis, *shen-men,* and blood-letting at ear apex.

Analysis: Our selection of acupuncture points is based on the discussions of the heart and kidney in the viscera theory of traditional Chinese medicine. According to the viscera theory, heart stores *shen* (spirit) and controls blood. The failure of heart to store *shen* is often caused by insufficient blood from the heart. As a result, the patient is accompanied by dizzy spells and headache. Kidney stores *ch'i* (energy), and its function is intimately related to that of the heart. When the "heart and kidney fail to communicate," a syndrome such as neurasthenia occurs. Again, because the "brain is the mansion of *yuan-shen* (original spirit or soul)" and controls spiritual activities, the acupuncture point of *shen-men* (spiritual gate) and dermis are thus selected to regulate the excitement and restraint functions of the cerebral cortex in order to attain a new balance between the two. Blood-letting at ear apex is effective for tranquilization and lowering pressure.

After the first insertion, the patient felt sleepy. After the second insertion, he slept for 4-5 hours. After two series of treatments, the patient slept for 6-7 hours every night, and worked energetically during the day. The syndrome of dizzy spells and headache was gone. He was very pleased with the ear acupuncture treatment.

Combination of Ear Acupuncture Points for Curing Otitis Media

Chang, female, age 19, an educated youth.

The patient complained about her two ears discharging pus since she was one year old and about her loss of hearing. For eighteen years, her two ears discharged pus which stank during the summer. After five treatments, purulency ceased and inflammation disappeared.

Selection of Acupuncture Points: kidney, outer ear, inner ear, internal secretion, and occiput.

Analysis: According to *The Yellow Emperor's Classic of Internal Medicine,* "Air from the kidneys is connected with the ears; thus, when there is harmony in the kidneys, ears can distinguish the five musical notes." The intimate relationship between kidneys and ears suggests that ear disease can be treated by strengthening kidneys, and so the kidney point is selected. The selection of the acupuncture points of the inner ear and outer ear is to produce impact on the affected areas, to build resistance, and to attain new balance. The selection of accupuncture points of occiput and internal secretion is for counteracting inflammation.

Combination of Ear Acupuncture Points for Curing Auditory Vertigo

Ts'ai, age 43, a female helper in a school.

The patient had a four-year pathological history. At the onset of disease, she could not raise her head and open her eyes, felt everything around her turn, and vomited continually. Sometimes, it lasted as long as several weeks. In August, 1970, the patient was struck by the syndrome again, and after three days of continual suffering, she received ear acupuncture treatment.

Selection of Acupuncture Points: kidney, occiput, inner ear, *shen-men*, and stomach.

Analysis: The three acupuncture points of *shen-men*, occiput, and stomach are selected to regulate the activities of the nerve center, to control dizzy spells, and to halt vomiting. Because the syndrome is usually caused by the malfunction of the labyrinth, the inner ear point is selected to treat the origin of the syndrome. According to traditional Chinese medicine, the "brain is the sea of marrow," and "air from kidneys reaches ears," there are intimate relationships between the kidneys and brain and between kidneys and ears. In the course of treatment, since the kidney point was added, the effect was obviously enhanced.

After only three treatments, the patient could get up and walk around. After seven treatments, her syndrome was cured. We paid her a visit one year later, and the patient reported: "In the past the syndrome usually broke out several times a year, and since I underwent ear acupuncture treatment, it never occurred again."

Clinical Record of Curing Rheumatic Myocarditis

Wang, female, age 13, a worker's daughter at Maanshan.

When she was 8 years old, her two knee joints suffered aching pain, and her tonsils were often inflamed. When 10 years old, she was hospitalized for scarlet fever and was diagnosed as suffering from rheumatic myocarditis. Noise was detected at the frontal area of her heart during contraction, gallop rhythm, and irregular heart rhythm. The test showed anti-"0" 833 units and blood sedimentation rate around 40. The use of penicillin, gantrisin, and other medicines produced no curing effect. In September, 1969, an electrocardiograph test diagnosed sinus tachycardia at 130 beats per minute, premature contraction, and high blood pressure at the cardiac ventricle. The patient felt excessive heart beats and fatigue whenever the weather underwent a sudden change or she caught cold. In June, 1970, the patient's parents asked us to give her ear acupuncture treatment.

Selection of Acupuncture Points: heart, sympathetic, small intestine, spleen, dermis, and internal secretion.

Analysis: The purpose of selecting the three acupuncture points of the heart, sympathetic, and dermis is to regulate the function of the central nervous system, to strengthen the function of myocardium, and to improve circulation. The selection of internal secretion is to stimulate internal metabolism, to counteract rheumatism, and to build up resistance. According to the viscera theory that heart and small intestine are intimately related, the simultaneous use of the acupuncture points of the heart and small intestine will enhance the curing effect.

After four series of treatments, the patient felt a great improvement in her heartbeat. A laboratory test showed that anti-"0" 500 units and blood sedimentation rate normal. The electrocardiograph read sinus tachycardia at 97 beats per minute. Two more series of treatments were given for consolidating the cure. In early 1971 the patient went back to school.

Assessment of 28 cases of Tertian Malaria

Our unit treated 28 cases of tertian malaria with ear acupuncture. In 23 cases, blood smear examination showed Plasmodium positive. The other five cases all had a pathological history of recurrences for more than twice continually and showed typical clinical symptoms. Because of lack of facilities, no blood smear was prepared.

Selection of Acupuncture Points: liver, spleen, dermis, suprarenal gland, and internal secretion.

Analysis: Malaria is a disease of the netlike corium system. The life cycle of plasmodia in human body involves the liver and spleen, and in clinical examination syndromes such as hepatomegalia and splenomegalia are often detected. According to traditional Chinese medicine, prolonged malaria may cause a lump underneath the left ribs. In the course of treatment, the acupuncture points of the liver and spleen have an important function in turning plasmodia in blood corpuscles to negative. Therefore, in treating malaria we stress the acupuncture points of the liver and spleen. The purpose of selecting acupuncture points of suprarenal gland and internal secretion is to control the syndrome, to reduce fever, and to counteract hypersensitivity. The plasmodia in the process from multiplication in blood corpuscles to destruction of blood corpuscles causes hemolyzation which induces a series of reactions in organs, and so the acupuncture points of suprarenal gland and internal secretion have the function of controlling the syndrome. The acupuncture point of dermis is for tranquilization and reduction of fever.

In most cases, after 1-3 times of needle insertion, the disease is under control. Generally, after three treatments, the syndrome disappears, and a blood smear test two or three days later will show it negative. This will then be considered a cured case. If after three treatments the disease is still not under control, it will be considered a case of failure in statistics. The method is needle insertion once a day on the day of recurrence and one hour before recurrence, with no definite time table for needle insertion on the day of non-recurrence. The time for leaving the needle in place is about 2-3 hours. The net result of treating 28 of tertian malaria is that 24 have been cured and 4 remained uncured.

The curing rate is 85.7% (see Table 13-1) after 1-3 times of needle treatment, a clear indication of effectiveness in treating tertian malaria. Generally, drug treatment also takes 1-3 days or longer to cure. But if the disease is not under control after three needle treatments, the patient should be treated by other methods. The recommendation is made because one more recurrence will cause the patient more pain. Therefore, in order to improve the curing effect of ear acupuncture in treating tertian malaria more research is needed in selecting acupuncture points as well as in timing needle insertion.

TABLE 13-1
Comparison of Number of Needle Insertions and Curing Rate

| No. of Needle Insertions | Curing Rate | | | No Effect | Total |
	Once	Twice	Thrice		
No. of cases	8	9	7	4	28
percent (%)	28.6	32.1	25	14.3	100

A Discussion of
"Normal Sensitive Points"

The problem of whether there are "normal sensitive points" is often faced by those who study ear acupuncture and ear acupuncture diagnosis. In recent years, there have been controversies over "normal sensitive points." Based on numerous clinical cases, we offer our view of the problem.

When intestinal organs or external limbs suffer ailment or are injured, generally some abnormal phenomena will appear in the corresponding or representative areas of the auricle. Naked eyes can observe peeling or blood shooting or a papule at certain spots of auricular skin. If pressed with a probe, the spots will feel pain. If tested with an acoustic auricular acupuncture points locating device, they will transmit sound. We often use such reactions as a logical basis for diagnosis and treatment. But why when certain parts undergo pathological development, such reflective points will appear on the auricle? According to traditional Chinese medicine, acupuncture points are reflective points of air passing through vessels to reach surface, and ailing vessels and meridians obstruct circulation of air to incur pain. If there is disease in the lungs, the central chamber defies harmony. A passage in "Plain Dialogue: Enumeration of Pains" says "Meridians are channels for ceaseless circulation. When chill air invades the vessels, the circulation is slowed down or obstructed. If it resides outside the vessels, blood circulation becomes insufficient; if it resides in the vessels, air circulation is obstructed. The result is pain." That is to say, disease causes obstruction. On the basis of the above theory, pain phenomenon results from disease which causes obstruction of vessels and meridians in viscera and bowels, body, and the four limbs.

In recent years because of popularization and development of ear acupuncture treatment, a number of ear acupuncture points locating devices are designed on the basis of the phenomena of low electric resistance and high conductivity at auricular spots. The use of instrument to locate reflective points helps identify precise ear acupuncture points. Since the theory of appearance of reflective points has not been fully developed, in the course of exploration reflective points unrelated to disease are also located. As a result, some people call those ever present points normal sensitive points or "pseudo-*yang* points." In clinical diagnosis and treatment, the acupuncture points of the heart, liver, spleen, lung, and kidney often show sensitive reaction, but their corresponding organs do not necessarily have pathological development. We would never understand the phenomenon if we do not analyze it according to the viscera theory of traditional Chinese medicine.

Whether "normal sensitive points" exist must be discussed from the two aspects of technicality and the problem itself.

(1) Technical aspect: The appearance of many "reflective points" may be caused by a number of factors. These include hypersensitivity of the ear acupuncture points locating device, too much pressure applied when the ear is probed, excessive secretion of grease in triangular fossa, cavum concha, and cymba concha, too much perspiration at auricle because of summer heat, and low electric resistance in the case of people who work indoors year round. If naked eyes do not observe *yang* reactions such as skin peeling, discoloration, and deformation, or if no pain is felt when the spots are pressed with a probe, they cannot be used as evidence for treatment and supplementary diagnosis. These are technical problems.

(2) Theoretical aspect: Aside from reflective points which can be solved by technical improvement, there are some which appear to bear no relation to disease. For patient of tinnitus aurium or

deafness, not only his acupuncture points of the inner ear and outer ear but also his kidney, heart, and occiput points show reaction and feel pain when pressed, yet he does not suffer diseases of the urinary system and of the cardiovascular system. According to the viscera theory of traditional Chinese medicine, "the orifice of the kidney is the ear," "when kidneys are insufficient ears turn deaf," and "the secondary orifice of the heart is the ear." These passages explain the dialectical relations between the acupuncture points of the kidney and heart and tinnitus aurium. Clinical application also proves that when the acupuncture points of the heart and kidney are added in treating tinnitus aurium and deafness, the curing effect is enhanced.

According to one test, 78% of healthy people are sensitive at the kidney area of the auricle. We have done considerable research work on the kidney point which shows that the reflective point at the kidney area is related to diseases of the urinary and reproductory system, the internal secretion system, the nervous system, the skeletal system, and the five sense organs. In order to establish whether "normal sensitive points" exist, one Peking unit examined 60 air force pilots and found not a single sensitive point. This deserves our further exploration of the internal relationship between the acupuncture points and mutual assistance and mutual restraint of acupuncture points. We believe if at the present stage we identify a number of "normal sensitive points," it will more or less mislead us in diagnosis or treatment and also may be detrimental to the theoretical development of ear acupuncture. These are some preliminary observations, and correct understanding of the problem will depend on further scientific research and free discussion in medical and scientific circles.

A Discussion of Multiple Uses of the Same Acupuncture Point

Many people have difficulty in understanding why ear acupuncture can cure a large variety of diseases. We also have gone through a process from "not understanding" or "insufficient understanding" gradually to "understanding" or "better understanding."

In treating a case of chronic bronchitis with ear acupuncture, the patient told us that for five years he had completely lost his smelling ability, but that after a period of treatment he could smell the aroma of perfumed soap. At the same time, the color of vitiligo on his chest was turning from white to healthy red and the affected area was receding. We did not know that the patient also suffered chronic rhinitis and vitiligo. Why is it that in treating his chronic bronchitis, the other two diseases are also being cured?

What is the relationship between chronic bronchitis on the one hand and chronic rhinitis and vitiligo on the other? How they are mutually affected? After we examined references, reviewed the treatment record, and made a comparative study, we concluded that the result was attained by needling a primary acupuncture point—the lung—which was the key factor. The viscera theory of traditional Chinese medicine says: "the orifice of the lungs is the nose," "when there is harmony in the lungs the nose smells odors," and "lungs control skin and hairs all over the body." This "bonus" in treating the above case led to our new understanding of the acupuncture point of the lung. We thought if the acupuncture point of lung controls skin and hairs all over the body and is effective in curing vitiligo, can it be used for treating other skin diseases? Is this consideration realistic?

During a certain period, we treated five cases of urticaria and ten cases of neurogenic dermatitis with the lung as a primary acupuncture point in the combination and attained satisfactory results. We further used this acupuncture point broadly in treating other diseases of the same system, such as shingles, dermatophiliasis, eczema, tinea, and alopecia areata and attained very good results.

From the broad clinical application of the primary acupuncture point of the lung, we wondered whether other primary acupuncture points such as the heart, spleen, and kidney have similar characteristics. We then tested the acupuncture point of the kidney. For instance, in treating a leading cadre who suffered years of neurasthenia and could not sleep well, we used the kidney as the primary acupuncture point. In the process of treatment, as the patient's headache gradually disappeared and sleep improved, his loose teeth were also gradually consolidated. Why in treating neurasthenia, loose teeth were also unexpectedly cured? In fact, according to the viscera theory of traditional Chinese medicine, kidneys are related to bones, and this "unexpected cure" is effected by the acupuncture point of the kidney, for "kidneys control bones," "bones produce marrow," and "teeth are the residue of bones."

Thus, we further recognize the special, extremely subtle interrelationship between the ear and other parts of the body. Therefore, the function of ear acupuncture points is not limited to one point with one specific treatment effect, but each point having multiple uses. As a result, the scope of ear acupuncture is broadened and its effect enhanced.

We must follow Chairman Mao's teaching: "Traditional Chinese medicine is a great treasure house which must be further explored and enriched." We must explore the heritage of traditional Chinese medicine, use modern scientific method for research and development, expound the essence of traditional Chinese medicine and reasons for its curing effect, elevate it to the level of modern science, and apply it in clinical practice. Advanced work in this field is to be continued.

"Within the scope of struggle for production and scientific experiment, mankind makes constant progress and nature undergoes constant change; they never remain at the same level." We must follow Chairman Mao's teaching, "practice, knowledge, more practice, more knowledge," and continually try to understand the function of ear acupuncture points and to provide scientific explanations for ear acupuncture curing effects in order to open a new avenue for ear acupuncture treatment of common diseases, recurring diseases, and rare and difficult diseases.

APPENDIX **III**

Some Explanations for Pain Caused in Ear Acupuncture

We have been confronted with the problem of whether pain is unavoidable in needle insertion and whether the more painful the insertion, the better the cure. Numerous clinical applications prove that the ear is by no means a simple, isolated organ of hearing. It is intimately connected with all parts of the human body. Every intestinal organ, or every part of the body, has a "representative area" at the auricle. When an intestinal organ or a certain part of human body undergoes pathological development, a specific "pain point" appears in the specific "representative area." This specific "pain point" at the auricle is both the reflective point as well as the curing point of the disease.

In clinical practice, we witnessed this interesting phenomenon: a patient who suffered periodic gastric spasm had no "pain sense" at the stomach point of the auricle, or the "representative area" of the stomach, when his condition was normal. When his stomach suffered spasm, the point felt a clear burning pain. After this "representative area" was needled and spasm disappeared, the burning pain at the "representative area" was also gone. At the same time, we made this comparative study: when the patient's stomach had spasmodic stroke, the pain threshold at the "representative area" of the auricle lowered and clear pain was felt when needled. On the other hand, if the patient's condition was normal, using the same method to needle the same area caused no clear pain, or no pain at all, which showed its pain threshold was higher than during spasmodic stroke.

We believe that the appearance and disappearance of a pain point correspond to the appearance and disappearance of disease. Generally speaking, the milder the disease, the less painful the pain point; the severer the disease, the more painful the pain point. When disease is cured, the pain point disappears. When disease transfers from one organ to another, pain also shifts from one point to another. Therefore, the more accurate the pain point is located, the more effective the disease will be cured. Numerous clinical applications prove that pain in ear acupuncture is in direct ratio to curing effect. Since a pain reflective point itself is sensitive to pain, needling this point is more painful than the normal ear acupuncture point.

Whether the ear acupuncture point is correctly needled can be verified by the nature of pain. The pain caused by needling the correct acupuncture point is a continual burning pain or starting pain spreading from inside to outside. There is a sense of relief when the pain is over. If it is a general pain caused by needling, or by inserting the needle in the incorrect acupuncture point, it is only a kind of superficial pain, a skin level pain with short duration. There will be no sense of relief when the pain is over, and of course, no expected curing effect.

Furthermore, of those who received ear acupuncture treatment 95% feel a sense of "heat" and its transmission when the needle is inserted. Some patients feel heat at the head, others feel heat at the palm and bottom of the foot, others feel heat at the thorax, abdomen, and back, and still others feel heat transmitted throughout the entire body. We believe that this heat and its transmission can be the special needle reaction in ear acupuncture treatment and the key to cure. Whether a sense of heat is felt when the auricle is inserted with the needle is the criterion to determine the correctness of the acupuncture point (pain point). Only when the correct acupuncture point is needled will this sense of heat and heat transmission be produced.

There was a case of vasculitis. The patient's two pedi-dorsal arteries and right superior ulnary collateral artery had no pulse, the ailing limbs were pale and cold, and the toes of the right foot turned back. Before acupuncture treatment, he could not walk. After he underwent five series of treatments, his pulse returned, the complexion of his ailing limbs turned healthy red, and the toes of his right foot also turned healthy red. At first he limped and then he walked five *li* (1⅔ miles) without the support of crutches. In the course of treatment, each time the needles were inserted, the patient strongly felt transmission of heat. He could accurately tell where heat was transmitted when each needle was inserted.

The human body is a unified, organic whole. Under normal conditions, the activities of viscera, body, and limbs are in harmony. When an intestinal organ or a certain part of body undergoes pathological development, this balance is overturned. We think that the function of ear acupuncture treatment is that by needling specific "pain points," metabolism of the whole organic system is stimulated, all internal positive elements activated, and body resistance strengthened. We believe that the "heat" produced by needling pain points causes a good, active reaction of viscera and limbs, rearranges unbalance, regulates disharmonious organs, and establishes new balance. For instance, needling acupuncture points of the stomach and duodenum produces a certain amount of heat which leads to clear change in the secretion and motion functions of the digestive system, that is, increasing secretion of digestive juices and speeding up motion of the stomach and intestines to strengthen the resistance capacity of the organs and improve the condition of nourishment.

Pain caused by ear acupuncture in clinical application is a problem worthy of further research. A certain amount of pain is necessary and also effective. But thinking that the more painful the treatment the better is groundless. How to reduce or eliminate pain in ear acupuncture without effecting a cure is a problem yet to be resolved in clinical application.

Postscript

Following Chairman Mao's teaching, "Traditional Chinese medicine is a great treasure house which must be further explored and enriched," we collected data and compiled this booklet to meet the demand of the masses. In presenting our experience in ear acupuncture treatment for more than ten years, we hope, together with other medical personnel, to explore, compile, and study the theory of ear acupuncture in disease treatment and to grasp the rules of its function. We hope ear acupuncture will play a greater role in clinical treatment of workers, peasants, soldiers, in promoting and enriching traditional Chinese medicine, and in developing a new unified medical and pharmaceutical science in new China.

In the course of writing and editing *Ear Acupuncture*, we once again received education in the two-road struggle between historical materialism and historical idealism, between materialism and idealism, and between dialecticism and metaphysics. The fundamental difference of the two-road struggle in medical and health work is whether medical work should be guided by the proletarian world outlook or by the bourgeois world outlook. The likes of Liu Shao-ch'i basically denied the importance of practice in medical treatment as objective reality, spread reactionary view of "medical mysticism," shouted absurd slogans such as "traditional Chinese medicine is unscientific," and "acupuncture and moxibustion kill pain but do not cure diseases." Essentially, they believe that knowledge was inherited, and rejected that knowledge originated in practice and was a reflection of the objective world. If we do not study the proletarian world outlook and do not repudiate the bourgeois world outlook, medical science cannot be advanced. The process of writing and editing *Ear Acupuncture* has been for us also a process of learning, a process of repudiating erroneous views. As we do not have profound knowledge of Marxism, Leninism, and Mao Tse-tung Thought and insufficient accumulation of clinical experiences, many of our views are rather unrefined. There must be shortcomings and mistakes in this book, and we sincerely hope to have the benefit of valuable comments from medical personnel and the public.

In the preparation of this volume, we received assistance from a number of agencies. The Medical Instrument Section of Nanking Electric Tube Factory provided us with their experience of designing and testing ear acupuncture points locating devices. Shenyang Medical College supplied us with pictures of the distribution of auricular nerves and blood vessels as well as written material. We also received considerable support from the General Hospital of the People's Liberation Army, Shanghai Traditional Chinese Medicine Research Institute, and Shanghai Municipal June 26th New Acupuncture Treatment Clinic. All the assistance which enriches the content of this booklet is hereby acknowledged.

The *Ear Acupuncture* Editorial
Team of An Army Unit in Nanking
November 1972

Afterword

In the following pages, Dr. Frank Z. Warren, executive director of the National Acupuncture Research Society, describes the application of ear acupuncture techniques to ameliorate drug withdrawal symptoms. The work stands as a dramatic testimonial for ear acupuncture.

A counter to drug reaction and withdrawal symptoms has been made possible by a new approach which involves the ear at two points. Combining the techniques of American and Chinese physicians in this instance provides a perfect example of a bridge between the Eastern and Western worlds of medicine.

This approach was first attempted as a result of a serendipitous discovery made in Hong Kong at the Tung Wah and Kwong Wah hospitals. The doctors involved in the Orient were H. L. Wen and S. Y. C. Cheung from the Neurosurgical Unit of the Kwong Wah Hospital in Kowloon; and in the U.S., Drs. Lester Sacks and Timothy Smith.

Normally, the approach to drug treatment is as unsatisfactory in China as in this country. Two avenues are usually utilized; one, the psychiatric-psychotherapy route, which would include group therapy, social or milieu pressure therapy, aversion therapy, and hypnotic therapy. It would emphasize the alleviation of dependency factors and other psychotherapeutic support systems.

The other approach, strictly physical, would embrace chemical replacement therapy (methadone for heroin, dilantin for phenobarbital, etc.) and withdrawal therapy (not really therapy). In advanced programs both methodologies have been employed. However, with the advent of acupuncture as a world phenomenon, rather than as an Oriental curiosity, another possibility seems imminent and practical.

Mainly it involves acupuncturing three times daily, using two small needles placed at the bottom of the shell-like concha of both ears. The technique seems spectacularly efficient for many reasons. For one thing, a general tonification with acupuncture seems to be one of the more noteworthy contributions toward alleviating the depression factor found in many dependency profiles. Other advantages are that the method is very cheap, very simple, and will not produce debilitating side effects. It reduces the security problems of maintaining a clinic, yields quick results, seems to satisfy the patient not only as to the amelioration of his symptoms but in fact goes further in replacing the urge to take the drug. In the hospital the stay is frequently shortened. And, most importantly, there is no question of substituting one addiction (methadone) for another, as in most cases of physical-chemical replacement therapy.

Since the original study of 40 cases, many more studies have been instituted, in New York and Los Angeles. Thus far, the results are most promising, having produced a good response to the treatment in patients where the years of addiction were as high as 58!

The explanation for the description as a serendipitous discovery can be attributed to the fact that more than half the patients had been admitted with pulmonary complaints, mostly asthma, pulmonary tuberculosis, and emphysema. Others were admitted for the treatment of arteriosclerotic heart disease, tumor of the bladder, cor pulmonare, fractured legs, fractured skulls, rheumatism, low back pain, and others. The wide variety of primary complaints seems to augment the results obtained.

The original Wen technique is a modified technique quite easy to perform and not time-consuming. Present techniques develop more of a euphoria, which supports the psychiatric profile, and as it is now practiced involves needling the patient's ear subcutaneously for one-half centimeter in the middle of the concha. The "lung point" is used, since it is easily found and covers an area which really consists of two points. After the ear is cleansed with an alcohol sponge, a sterile acupuncture needle connected to an electric stimulator is inserted. Electric stimulation is gradually increased from 0 to 125 Hz., and the intensity is increased until the patient feels the flow of current but does not have any pain in his ear. If the patient complains of pain, the intensity of the current is diminished until the patient states he feels comfortable, and then gradually increased again to where a current of .2 to .4 milliamps is applied. Since drug addicts are notoriously sensitive, the electric stimulator must be utilized carefully, for the possibility of infection and tissue damage is high in the debilitated tissue one finds as a feature of most addicts.

In each case, the duration of the treatment varies on the individual, the drugs, and the length of time that drugs have been misapplied. The average stimulation varies from 15 minutes to 20 minutes, although treatments of 45 minutes are not uncommon. The patient is treated on days 1, 2, 3, 5, 7, 9, 12, 15, 18, and 21, spacing out the days in this manner as is required. If the complaints are plentiful, the schedule can be intensified, but an application somewhat similar to a withdrawal program can be utilized.

On the first few days, the patient is treated two or three times a day, followed by two stimulations for the next two or three treatments, and finally one stimulation on the final days. He may return for reinforcement ad lib.

Amelioration of the symptoms is usually obtained almost immediately, within 10 to 15 minutes. The aching and shivering may be the first symptoms to disappear, after which some of the abdominal "butterflies" will go away. The runny noses and eyes, and salivating mouths, may dry; and the headaches, nausea, and vomiting may disappear entirely. Breathing may return to normal and the patient may feel refreshed, relaxed, warm, and decidely less fearful.

Wen describes the effect as follows: "A sense of general well-being is described by all patients undergoing treatment. They feel less drowsy and much more interested in their surroundings than before, and they quickly gain an interest in conversation and reading. All report better appetite and easier bowel function. It is common to find the patients getting up and engaging in drinking tea or coffee and in eating a lot of cakes, bread, and noodles soon after the stimulation is over. Often during the stimulation the patients ask to go to the toilet to urinate, which suggests that this treatment may have a diuretic effect. All of these activities are in contrast to the patients' condition before the stimulation sessions, when they were invariably withdrawn and preferred to sleep fully dressed and covered from head to foot in bed. They then disliked food, some moaned with pain in the back or abdomen, while others had wheezing and coughing as well as the usual symptoms of withdrawal. Their main interest during that time was to know when the next stimulation would be given." [1]

Most times the patient indicated when the treatment was to end. The goal was to have the patient feel as relaxed and "satisfied" as if he had had a full dose of the drug he was addicted to. However, no attempt was made to equilibrate the euphoria derived from the drug.

In toto, it has been stated that 60 days are needed to restore the normal central nervous function after withdrawal.

Ear Acupuncture Stapling Procedure

The disadvantages of acupuncturing a group of addicts three times daily are obvious. Added to the medical problems are the difficulties in maintaining decorum in the doctor's office. In some instances, petty thievery becomes uncontrollable, a not inconsiderable item. In Los Angeles, a felicitous application of a surgical stapling machine devised by Russian scientists was developed. Originally intended to facilitate the placement of countless intestinal sutures, it was employed in a startling adaptation—stapling the addict's ears. As a more practical method of treatment, the stapling procedure far surpasses the original method described by Wen. The metallic stapler, with a standard SM-25 staple,

---

[1] *The Asian Journal of Medicine*

provides what might be called a "built-in acupuncturist".

The concept was to eliminate the necessity of an acupuncturist three times daily. By inserting a small device in the concha, the addict could stimulate manually to produce the desired effect. The physical construction of the staple lent itself well for this purpose. Not only was stimulation of the local "lung point" achieved, but activation of the "liver point" adjacent to it as well. The external stimulation was performed by the addict himself simply by moving the outer edge or exposed edge of the staple several times daily or when the "withdrawal syndrome" became difficult for the patient.

(1) With patient lying prone, 0.25 cc of 1 percent Xylocaine is injected through 27-gauge needle into ear concha approximately 0.5 cm from the external auditory canal orifice, raising the skin from the cartilage. This procedure is repeated bilaterally.

(2) With the stapler partially "cocked" so that the SM-25 staple is exposed, the staple is placed in a 45 degree rotation allowing puncture of the "lung" and "liver" regions of the ear points. Again this is repeated bilaterally.

(3) An antibiotic treatment such as neosporin is used for local application to the areas, to reduce chance of cellulitis and secondary infection.

(4) The patient is instructed in the use of the ointment and the fingertip stimulation of the staple. They are further advised to return at weekly intervals to evaluate the staple puncture effect.

Utilizing this method, Dr. Lester Sacks of Los Angeles has treated approximately 200 patients in a control environment and achieved the following startling results to date. Approximately 34 percent have been drug-free for three months. All addicts received some amelioration of their symptoms and some reduction of their drug intake, with the exception of 15 percent, who were stapled but did not return for follow-up evaluation. The reduction of a drug such as methadone, for example, was tabulated as from 20 milligrams to 5 milligrams in seven to ten days; in other words, a reduction of 75 percent of their intake in less than a fortnight. Although these results are premature, the benefit of stimulating the ear "lung point" in addiction therapy seems strongly indicative.

Index